DANIEL SWIFT

DIARY
OF A FORMER
FAT MAN

*My real world year-long journey
from obesity to a healthier
weight and lifestyle*

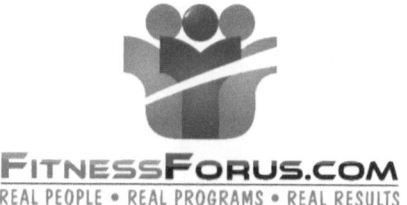

FitnessForus.com
REAL PEOPLE • REAL PROGRAMS • REAL RESULTS

ISBN: 1453732470
ISBN-13: 9781453732472

Visit www.createspace.com to order additional copies.

This book is dedicated to all those who are also battling weight loss after years of obesity just like I did. Remember, if I can do it you can too!

My wife deserves a special thank you. I may never know why you love me but I thank God everyday that you do. Love you, my CPITA.

CONTENTS

Chapter One: How It All Began 1

Chapter Two: Act One... 5

Chapter Three: An Unplanned Hiatus 63

Chapter Four: Act Two.. 69

Chapter Five: Lessons Learned; Act Two 117

Chapter Six: Act Three 119

Chapter Seven: Lessons Learned; Act Three and This Year 193

CHAPTER ONE

HOW IT ALL BEGAN

"Well, you didn't have a heart attack." As relieved as I was to hear the emergency room doctor say that, the look of shock on his face did throw me a bit. I guess it is typical for an obese smoker close to forty showing up with chest pains to be suffering a heart attack. Well, it wasn't a heart issue. It turns out I had developed a chronic stomach condition that simulates a heart attack—lucky me. This was a real wake-up call that forced me to take a hard look at my health.

I decided, for the first time in my life, to get my weight under control. In the past, I had given half-hearted attempts to drop some pounds but this time was different. I really felt like I was battling for my life. The years of excess weight and poor health had really begun to take a toll on the quality of my life. Having never really given my health a second thought, I found a sea of information and programs that promised to shed weight quick and painlessly. I quickly realized most of these programs were nothing but empty promises. I then went to the basics of weight loss: consume fewer calories than I use, combining a low calorie diet with exercise.

To fulfill my strategy I first picked a popular prepackaged meal plan, which limited my intake to 700 to 1000 calories a day of bars, shakes, and one regular meal a day. There are a host of programs like this on the market; basically they work by controlling portions, having you eat on a regular basis, and limiting the total calories. I picked this type of plan because not only would it take weight off quickly, it would also provide time for my body and mind to reset the way I look at food. After seventy-plus days, I no longer craved a lot of the things that had made me obese. I educated myself about making healthy food selections (although as you will see, I will always have a weak spot for pizza).

After this first stage, I experimented with ways to incorporate more real foods into my options while still taking off weight. This proved a lot harder than the prepackaged menu but, by the end of the year, I really had it down and was able have a diet of real food as I continued to lose weight. The problem with the prepackaged food plans is that once you go off them, the weight comes flooding back on, so I wanted to design a long-term healthy eating plan utilizing real foods that tasted good and still promoted weight loss. Even after the year detailed here was up, I continued to enjoy this real foods plan as I lost unwanted weight.

During this process I also got a real education on exercising, learning a lot of hard lessons about what not to do along the way. My naturally obsessive personality resulted in endless hours spent researching exercise and healthy eating. This culminated in me becoming certified in personal training and establishing fitnessforus. com as a free resource for those looking to lose weight and get healthy.

I spent the first twenty years of my adult life obese, to be honest, as I started this journey I couldn't remember not being fat. The most I ever weighed is 364 pounds; for most of the past twenty years the scale has rarely settled under 300 pounds. As I began, I despised exercise and my eating habits were horrible. I was a late-night gorger and avoided most foods with any real health benefits in favor of sweet treats and lard-laden options. Essentially I am the average obese American. Added to this I have a host of existing injuries and aches and pains in my ankles, knees, back, and shoulders.

Like many of my fellow obese Americans, I pay my mortgage by spending most of the day on my butt in front of a computer. This is a real program, done in real life; I didn't go away for six months to a fat camp, nor did I spend thousands of dollars or resort to any sort of surgery. Everything I did fit within the confines of the time restraints most of us circling forty with careers and family have.

What follows didn't start out as a book; it started out as a journal for me to vent. Believe me, I needed it, considering the massive changes ahead of me. My decision to share the journey was the result of friends and colleagues inquiring about how I achieved the results. What follows is my journey: mistakes, weight, measurements, and all. I hope it provides some help. If nothing else, realize that if I can do this, you can too!

CHAPTER TWO

ACT I

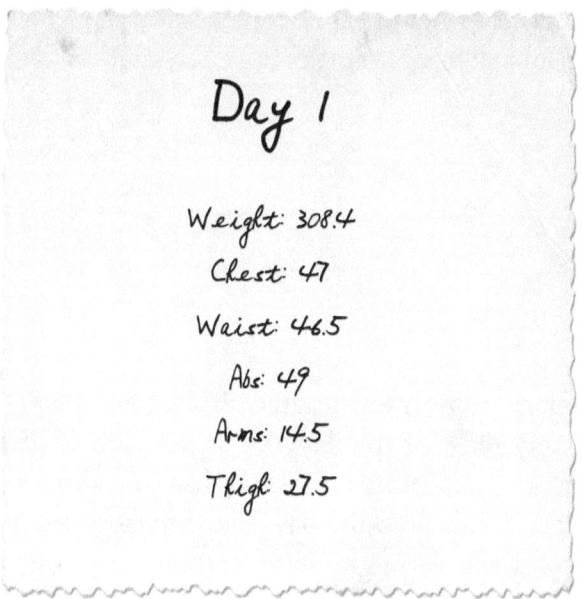

Day 1

Weight: 308.4
Chest: 47
Waist: 46.5
Abs: 49
Arms: 14.5
Thigh: 27.5

Seeing the scale over that three hundred number is bad; seeing it settle so comfortably over three hundred is much worse. I did eat myself sick yesterday, figured might as well go out with a bang. The packaged diet program I am on consists of five shakes or bars a day followed by six ounces of grilled chicken breast and a salad with light oil and vinegar dressing for dinner. So reading this isn't as boring as my eating, just assume that's all I ate on any given day unless I say otherwise.

I have typically preferred to save my eating for late-night power sessions. The sun goes down and my mouth is open for business, so eating first thing in the morning was a struggle, even though it was a minimal amount of food. I drank a lot of water today, more than I think I have drunk in years, and ate every two to three hours. Then, around 4 o'clock the headache hit. I took a couple migraine pills & it was gone in half an hour. So I enjoyed a diet soda over the next couple hours. I think all the water this program recommends drinking made the soda last longer. Before I began this program wouldn't drink sixty-four ounces of water a month. Doing it in one day is a lot tougher than I thought it was going to be. Day one wasn't the worst. The diet was better than I expected, the water was a lot tougher than I expected, but all in all feeling pretty good after day one.

Day 2

Another glorious morning began with a bar & a couple cups of coffee. Felt okay most of the day, did a good job of getting the full sixty-four ounces of water in, which has forced me to schedule a lot more pee breaks into the day. Had a massive headache around 3 PM; after a couple migraine pills, though, it went away. Never thought I would look forward to grilled chicken & a lettuce & cucumber salad. Seriously shocked by how excited this fat man gets over that combo.

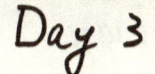

I woke up really easily this morning—guess when you take stuffing your face out of the nightly routine you sleep a bit better. One thing I have noticed is all the food commercials on TV, especially late at night. It's like they are saying, "Dan, we know you are on a diet & we know you're suffering through the highest level of temptation during the evening, so let's see if we can blitz your brain & break you, pork chop." Well, so far I haven't broken; of course I am only seventy-two hours into it so I wouldn't exactly call that evidence of my iron will. Nice increase in energy today, really noticeable. Hopefully that keeps up, as I will need all the energy I can get.

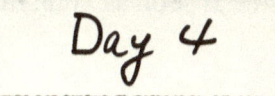

Okay, today the energy increase was really noticeable. From rise to shine I felt one hundred percent better than I have in years, & it's only day four! Even had the energy today to run to the hardware store & pick up paint & supplies to finally paint my home office, a project I have talked about but done little else about over the past six months. Today I did a little online research & discovered the BMI index. Based on this measure I should weigh 200 pounds, which means I started this diet being 108 pounds overweight! That's like a whole eighth grader! Now happily married and heading towards forty, I don't really have any desire to look like an underwear model. I would be happy to be just overweight, rather than obese. So I don't know how close I will get to that 200 number but time will tell.

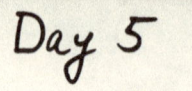

Day 5

Woke up with a ton of energy today & it carried through the day. So far the self-induced dietary restrictions seem to be worth the pain. Painted the office today, really broke a sweat. The work went well; not perfectly, but I am just happy to finally have the energy to do it. I guess I should consider myself making progress since I can see myself moving from fat & lazy to fat but not so lazy. I have to admit the increased activity—i.e. time I am not sitting on my butt—really kicked up my hunger. I have a fine tradition of rewarding any home improvement project with pizza. Oh & did I mention we were watching the hockey playoffs tonight? Another reason for pizza. But nope, I resisted; instead, had another helping of grilled chicken & salad. I made it through the night & went to bed filled with pride rather than pizza. Now I only have to convince myself that pizza isn't as satisfying as pride. Will let you know as soon as I pull that off.

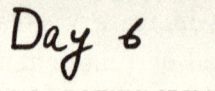

Day 6

Almost a week; almost time to jump on the scale. Well, not jump—I don't think the scale was built for that kind of impact. I am praying I see the scale under 300 pounds on Monday. Yeah, I know that is a lot to ask out of one week, but come on. I am starting at a huge weight & have made a dramatic change, so the results should be equally dramatic right? If I see the scale has only moved two pounds it's going to hard to stick with it, even though I feel better. I spent most of the day recovering from painting-related joint pain, a lovely side effect of being obese.

Day 7

It's a Sunday, so I slept in. Today should be the easiest day to stick with the program, since tomorrow is scale day. Spent the day hiding out in the house to avoid food temptation; hopefully I don't have to do that too much longer. Otherwise, I might be thinner, healthier, & crazier from fighting off the endless amount of food temptation the outside world throws at you constantly. Keeping my fingers crossed that tomorrow when I wake up I am rewarded with a sub-three hundred-pound figure on the scale. That just may make the last week all worth it. Otherwise I might as well have responded to the daily pizza place emails I get, being a frequent online customer in my former life as a fat man. Seriously, do they need to email me *every* day? I have to figure out how to unsubscribe. One ad had me ready to lick my computer screen. Nice job, marketing department.

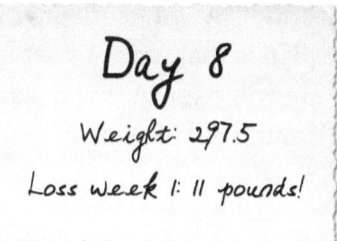

Day 8
Weight: 297.5
Loss week 1: 11 pounds!

Oh yeah!! Scale now comfortably settles under the three-hundred-pound mark! I couldn't be happier. Nicest of all: some shirts I haven't been able to wear in a while fit. I was so excited! I couldn't wait to go to the office for a meeting with the guy who convinced me to go on this diet in the first place—well, more accurately, his thirty-pound weight loss & noticeably increased energy from this program sold me. What has surprised me is how supportive my wife is. Not because she isn't normally supportive, but because she's naturally thin but has given up sweets & snacks to make my life a little easier. The support of those around you is very important; if we had a host of snacks in the house my life would suck a lot worse.

Day 9

Okay, today was a tough day. I don't know if it was because I had to deal with getting a new phone once my pit bull puppy chewed up mine but I was tempted to break all day. Somehow I made it through, perhaps by drinking so much water that there wouldn't have been room for food anyway. Maybe I need to watch less TV. The endless flow of good-looking food is killing me. Since I did lose 11 pounds last week I thought it would be easier to keep on the program; not so today. I am hoping the next week puts me in the 290-range, but that seems like a lot to ask after shedding 11 pounds in the first week. My plan is that, once I start to plateau, which everything I read tells me will happen, I can start to mix in exercise and hopefully push through the plateau.

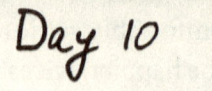

Day 10

A couple friends started this program & haven't made it past day one without wandering off it. I feel for them; the first few days are rough. Today was actually a pretty good day for me; I can see 290 at my next weigh-in. I am really getting use to the bars & shakes and most of the day I am just fine. The only time I have any real issues is late at night, my favorite time to eat. Had a ton of energy today, which is good thing, since it takes a lot of energy to move 297 pounds. Trying to guess how much I should expect to lose: my best guess is another 8 to 9 pounds this week to put me under 290; then the following week I should be in the low 280s; & then its two more weeks & I should be at 275. I haven't seen 275 in a long, long time, so I am curious to see what it looks & feels like.

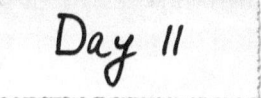

Day 11

Today was a weird day. My wife went to an awesome little pizza place we found right before I went on this program. Obviously, I wasn't in attendance. Pizza is a huge favorite of mine, so there is no way I could be around it & maintain both this program & my sanity. With the weigh-in just a few days away, I want to see that scale under 290 more than I want pizza. I went to a movie today & managed to not order any of the tempting candy. Halfway through the movie I munched on a bar, yum, yum. My energy is still way up. I couldn't get to sleep last night but I popped right out of bed nice & early this morning with no problem. Also was able to skip the coffee; I just didn't need it—first time in a long time I could say that. It is important to have small manageable milestones to celebrate while you work toward a long-term goal, so I am focused on the 290 number. We will see if I am right based on how well I stick with the program.

Day 12

Another relatively painless day all things considered. The only real torture was the endless number of TV commercials showing me all that I can't eat. I could, of course, turn the TV off, but my own thoughts of what I can't eat might be much worse. I have noticed I seem to be a bit on edge, a little quicker to lose my temper. I think that's just a side effect from depriving myself of the foods I love for the first time in thirty-seven years. I did manage to make my way through mowing the lawn today in about forty-five minutes, a personal best. I can really feel the positive effects of the diet and weight I have already lost.

Day 13

Another pretty tough day: it's a Saturday, which turned into a "run around to different stores like any typical suburban couple" day. Driving past all the fast-food places is like a gauntlet & somehow I made it through. Went through a bunch of the shirts that haven't fit in a while & now they do—pretty awesome; nice to see real noticeable results. When a three-hundred-pound man drops twenty pounds, it's good progress but doesn't make much of a dent in what you see in the mirror so it is nice to see some measurable results.

Day 14

I made it through painting the exercise room in record time; it really is so much easier to move around a smaller version of me. It's about the third time I have been in that room: the first two were to carry equipment into it. It was a bit easier this weekend to make it through the post-painting process without ordering pizza. They ought to make it harder to order food that's bad for you; I mean, you can order pizza from any number of places online & have it delivered, so really the only effort is answering the door. Tried some new chicken the past couple days, these little handy packages of six ounces of precooked seasoned chicken. They were pretty good just tossed on top of my romaine lettuce & cucumber salad & hit with a bit of light dressing. Not bad price either: $2.50 a pack, so you can have your food precooked & ready to go for under twenty bucks a week. Tomorrow is weight day. I am praying the scale is under 290 tomorrow; if it's not then I might just have to curl up in the fetal position with a pizza & comfort myself.

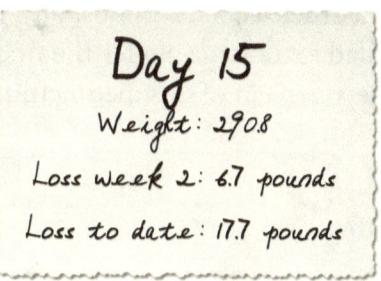

Day 15
Weight: 290.8
Loss week 2: 6.7 pounds
Loss to date: 17.7 pounds

Okay, so the scale wasn't under 290 as I hoped, dreamed, & prayed it would be, but I can't complain about losing almost eighteen pounds in fourteen days. My clothes are starting to fit a lot better at this point. I am a bit worried that the weight loss will keep declining, which will make it increasingly harder to stay with the program. Today I could have used a pizza, since I had to deal with the IRS. That's a stress that usually ends with a pizza, right? They were a lot nicer and easier to deal with than I expected but still a pizza-worthy moment. Instead, I took out the stress on my yard, putting in a good couple of hours of yard work & obliterating the poor shrubs hanging around my house.

Day 16

For some reason this was just a tough day to stick to the program and I have no idea why. It wasn't a particularly stressful day; in fact, it was relatively uneventful. Maybe my body is finally saying, "Hey, I am starving! Toss a pizza down your throat or I will punish you!" Or maybe it's all in my head. Most likely it's my mind not being able to figure out why I would suddenly start depriving myself of my beloved food after a solid thirty-seven years of following a "if it tastes good don't just eat it order seconds" philosophy. I pounded water all day & made my salad extra large. So far the first sixteen days have taught me that ninety percent of this dieting thing is purely mental.

Day 17

All right, I need to get out the house & do something fun before my head explodes. One of the advantages of being self-employed is being able to blow off a weekday from time to time. We toured an aircraft carrier ship, went through a submarine, & climbed into a fighter plane. Even though 290 still puts me in the obese category, I can really feel the difference. Took a bar & had lunch in about twenty seconds walking from the aircraft carrier to the sub. One of the nice things about the program is getting able to eat quickly on the run. Of course, one of the bad things about the program is not being able to sit down & make a pig out of myself, so I guess there are trade-offs.

Day 18

These late teen days are rough. My running theory is that the program is no longer new enough to be a novelty, but not yet established enough to be a habit, so life sucks in limbo. I did sneak onto the scale today: down to 287. I am right near my wedding weight. I took the four months before my wedding to get from 310 to 285. I lost that weight by working out five days a week, including an hour of cardio, & trying to eat healthy. A diet makes a much bigger impact than exercise & that "trying" to eat health & *actually* eating healthy are so not the same thing. Trying to stay motivated is getting harder; as time goes on, the weight will be dropping in smaller & smaller numbers, which will make it even harder.

Day 19

Another tough day for really no reason. Again I think it's just the late-teen limbo days. I had a hard time getting to sleep last night; I don't know if it's because I am craving the good old days of late-night gorging or because I have so much more energy without really increasing my activity level. The next thing that will spike my weight loss will probably be adding exercise. Simply walking for thirty minutes a day should make a big impact, since I have been so sedentary for so long. It's Friday & I had to turn down an invitation to go to the local nightclubs. That sucks. Here is the thing: I know I couldn't deal with the temptation of sitting around a bunch of people drinking what I am not allowed to & eating what I am not allowed to. At this point I am neither strong enough to resist the temptation nor down enough weight to allow for a temporary reprieve from the program, so it was a quiet Friday at home for me.

Day 20

Saturday. There's not much going on. I declined going to a couple places since not only would there be food there, but I would have to drive past food to get there, so again another day hiding in the house from the evils of temptation. I need to develop stronger willpower to be able to live a regular life again. Hell, I went out more when I was over 300 pounds & at that weight it was hard to move. I do have a fear that I am going to get stuck in the 285-range. That is why I have to throw exercise into the mix next week. That way I can hopefully jumpstart the weight loss & get into the unchartered territory that is the 270s. It was smart to make Monday scale day, because it makes it a little easier to get through the temptation-filled weekend, knowing that in a couple days I have to get my fat butt on a scale again.

Day 21

Sundays, you got to love Sundays. Still struggling with sleeping; maybe once I throw some light exercise into the routine the sleep issues will go away. I went & got coffee with the wife. It was the first time I had been in a coffee shop in three weeks. See, you might be shocked, but I prefer the creamy, rich & thick, thousand-calorie coffee shop drinks. However, today I had a regular cup of coffee, which has a lot fewer calories at a lot lower cost. Hey, you've got to celebrate the small things. Afterward we hit the grocery, & I managed to resist any urge to sample the food they were peddling. Whose idea was that anyway? The last thing I need is some pusher sitting on the corner of the isle offering what I don't need. So twenty-one days in & I am adjusting to the program. Not well enough to go to a restaurant but much better than I was during those teen days. If you go on this type of program, you better warn everyone around you that you will be a bit of a bear for a while—& not the fun cuddly teddy bear. There is something to the jolly fat person stereotype: as I get less fat I seem to be less jolly.

Day 22

Weight: 284.4

Loss week 3: 6.4 pounds

Loss to date: 24 pounds

Chest: 44.5, loss 2.5 inches

Waist: 44, loss 2.5 inches

Abs: 47, loss 2 inches

Arms: 14, loss .5 inch

Thigh: 27, loss .5 inch

I am under 285; not much under but it's something. Yeah I am still fat, but twenty-four pounds less fat than I was twenty-one days ago. Today was an incredibly easy day to stay on the program; it might have something to do with hitting that 285 milestone. Started walking today: I just spent thirty minutes at a quick pace through my neighborhood, and it's amazing how quickly the thirty minutes goes by. All right, so what have I learned in the first three weeks, or the first twenty-four pounds? First, if you are married you need a supportive spouse to make this program bearable. Second, you need to be very dedicated to it, because there are going to be plenty of days that suck. The dedication has to be there to keep at it. The third thing needed, at least for me, is the time to focus on making this a habit. Basically I spend most of my free time the first three weeks caved up in my house, which is what I needed to do make it through it. The fourth thing I have learned is that milestones are key; that's what will keep you moving along on tough days, not focusing on the eighty-plus pounds you want to take off, but rather that short distance milestone of ten pounds or so. The last key is having an endgame. I mean, let's be honest, there is no way some-one who loves food like I do wants to be on this program for the rest of my life. I foresee a day where I am in decent shape, have a good exercise routine, look & feel good, & can enjoy indulgent food from time to time while eating healthy most of the time.

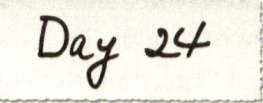

A pretty easy day: got my second walk in. Yeah, two points make a trend, right? Okay, maybe I am stretching it a bit. The sleep thing is still a struggle; I have a hard time getting to bed at what resembles a decent hour. Other than that I think I am on track. I am hoping the walking keeps the weight loss rolling at a good click. What may hold me back is my sedentary lifestyle. Let's just say I spend more hours on my butt than on my feet, so I am going to have to figure out a way to change that to keep the scale moving down.

Day 24

Another day, another walk. Now, if three points make a trend so three days of walking must make me a walker right? I added some-thing new to the salad & chicken combo I have enjoyed the past twenty-three days: fresh tomatoes. Oh yeah! At least it's something a little different. Even people in prison get some variety in their din-ing options.

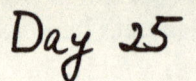

Day 25

Today's walk was a painful one. Between the knees & ankles hurting & the torn-up feet, it's no wonder more fat people don't walk. I can't believe I am still so fat. The weight that has come off is impressive, yeah, but I still have so much more to go. It's a stumbling block: you feel & look a lot better but when you look at how much more you have left to lose it seems impossible and makes you want to call it a day. Somehow I have to muster up the whatever you muster up to pull through this entire process.

Day 26

Had to take the wife to the airport early, so I got up at 5:30 AM, which totally screwed up my eating schedule. I stayed on the program but had to space out the meals a lot more because I know myself well enough to know I am not hitting the sheets early. No walk today; there was no way I could do it. I struggled to fall asleep last night because of the pain in my knees, so I figured I would give them a rest. Went & had a meeting over coffee & stuck to the regular coffee, no sweet & creamy frappe lardass for me. Hoping to keep it up & stay on track for 250 pounds in the next nine weeks before I return to Southern California for a wedding, my first trip out there since I moved almost a year ago. That should really shock people who haven't seen me in a year.

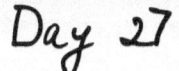

I checked my progress on the scale today: 282, only 2.4 pounds down, damn. I wanted to be under 280 by Monday & now I don't see that happening. I just can't see two-plus pounds coming off in the next two days. I did walk again today; figured I could stand the pain to make up for the fact that I am not losing weight at the pace I want to. If I slow down to two to three pounds a week, it's going to take forever to get less fat & I won't hit my 250 goal in time. I did start eating more precooked chicken; I don't think that could have anything to do with it though. I will see where I am Monday & make the changes I think will work, which is nothing but a guess, & then see where I am the following week. The last time I weighed myself early in the week I was motivated by the loss; now I am motivated by the slower loss, so I guess either way it can work as motivation.

Day 28

So I have been looking over everything to try to figure out why the weight loss has slowed down. I added walking this week, which may not seem like much but it's a zillion times more activity than normal, so if anything the weight loss should have picked up. I went through my food log & everything was in line: I ate every two & a half to three hours & I didn't break from the program. Okay so what could it be? My sleep has been off because my wife has been out of town & I hate sleeping alone, so instead I slept on the couch downstairs with the TV on & my dog at my feet. However, I did get five to six hours, which is pretty normal for me so I don't think that's it. Finally, I took a second look at my food log and discovered a couple things. First, I added tomatoes to my salad. I checked and tomatoes are in the high-carbohydrate category. Something told me, though, that tomatoes can't be the only problem so I kept digging. About eight days ago I switched my dressing, from light zesty Italian to light honey mustard. I figured light dressing is light dressing right? WRONG! It turns out the delicious honey mustard dressing has more than five times the amount of calories as the Italian I had been using! The honey mustard also has five grams of fat, which is five more than the Italian, & ten grams of carbohydrates, versus three for the Italian. Oh, & if that isn't enough, the honey mustard has eight grams of sugar compared to two for the Italian. No wonder so many of us are fat: even when we try to eat healthy they screw us. It couldn't be my fault for being too stupid or lazy to flip the bottles over & compare the two before throwing the bad one down my throat, could it? The honey mustard, it turns out, is light in comparison to their regular fat-filled & calorie-rich honey mustard. So it's off to the store for more zesty Italian. It is the Sunday before Memorial Day; what better to do than go to a grocery? As I walked my normal neighborhood route I turned down a couple offers for a free beer & a "regular" meal. By regular, of course, I mean they type of meal I enjoyed while climbing the fat charts up to 308 pounds. I had my nightly grilled chicken salad, this time with zesty Italian dressing—boy, do I miss the honey mustard—& passed out on the couch.

Day 29

Weight: 278.6

Loss week 4: 5.8 pounds

Loss to date: 29.8 pounds

I have no idea how that happened! I was assuming it would be like 280 or 281. It's amazing that I was able to shed thirty pounds in four weeks! I have never been a successful dieter; for me the rare times I had the thought of getting into shape I always opted to work out, as a man who has spent most of his adult life in the 300-pound range, I am rather naturally strong, so throwing weights around was always a lot more fun than counting calories & depriving myself. This is the single greatest weight loss feat of my thirty-seven years. All my clothes now fit nicely & next week, once I am under 275 pounds, I can move my fat clothes—the ones I bought after the scale climbed over 300 pounds—into the guest bedroom closet! I love the idea of clothes being too BIG for me; most of my life the opposite has been the case. This gives me the feeling that I might actually hit my goal of 250 in the next seven weeks! I have been thinking a lot lately about what my idea of "in shape" is. I am not a twenty-year-old guy trying to get a washboard stomach so I can make it onto an MTV reality show. So while my short-term goal remains the same—250 in the next seven weeks to shock the hell out of some of my friends in California—my long-term goal is open to change. I still think 225 would be ideal, but I could be wrong. I might be happy at 235 or, hell, maybe I won't be happy until I am 215. Only time will tell. I rather enjoyed my walk today, even though after three days straight my knees & ankles aren't happy.

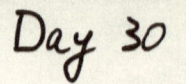

Day 30

"Oh my gosh, your head shrank!" This is what my wife said when I picked her up at the airport after her five-day trip. Kind of an odd thing to hear. What she meant is my face is so much thinner: I have a jaw line that is starting to appear & my chins are less massive. Even my eyes look wider since there is less cheek fat to fill the void. Maybe in another seven weeks when I return to California & see some people I haven't seen in almost a year, who rarely saw me under three hundred pounds, I might hear, "Wow were you fat," or, "I didn't know what the hell was under all that!" Either way, at least they won't be advising me to get my affairs in order & giving me directions to the closest cardiac ward.

Today was an off day from walking in my three days on, one day off schedule. I need the day to rest the knees & ankles. At forty, I find the joints need recovery time & the back goes out way too quickly & what the hell is that pulsing pain in my knees? So my advice to those in the sub-thirty-range is lose the weight now before the light amount of exercise you begin to introduce into your life kicks your butt in ways you can't even fathom. You have to listen to your body; if you can only handle walking three times a week I am sure it is more cardio then you have done the past decade.

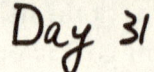

Day 31

Well, I cleared the month mark. Today was one of the tough days. Based solely on my own experience I have surmised the following: because your body is almost starving from its under one-thousand-calorie daily intake, which clearly will be a dramatic decrease for anyone who needs this program, & you've newly added exercise, there will be some days when your body gets angry at you. Today was one of those days. The effects have included light-headedness, odd aches & pains, upset stomach, & assorted levels of headaches. I stuck to the program & even got my scheduled walk in, even though I felt like crap the entire day.

Day 32

Bounced back nicely today after a tough day yesterday; actually, to-day was a breeze. I pounded through four hours of yard work, did a ton of work, & even managed to get my walk in. I don't know why today was so different than yesterday; maybe my body figures I am not going to listen to it so it might as well go with the program. My attitude was great today, couldn't have felt better. I will say the yard work was rather enjoyable. It started with simply cutting the grass, something that used to wipe me out by itself, but I moved on to weeding. Next thing I know I was removing every weed from my property & giving the house a great edge where the concrete meets the grass, all by hand. Got to say the extra energy and moving around thirty fewer pounds comes in handy.

Day 33

So I snuck onto the scale today for one of my unscheduled weigh-ins. The verdict: 275.8! The four hours of sweating through lawn work paid off. As someone who has spent the lion's share of the past couple decades doing very little physical activity, I must say the lawn work took its toll. I have a pain in my right knee that's just unbelievable. Add in the sore hands, shoulders, & back, and any movement is a bit rough right now. So I decided to make this my day off from walking. Hey, we all have to listen to our bodies, especially when they're screaming at us. Found some new zero-calorie honey Dijon salad dressing at the grocery today. Got to say it was pretty good—not as good as that calorie-packed "lite" honey mustard I had been enjoying, but an acceptable substitute.

Day 34

I got back to walking today despite my knee still hurting. You have to be able to tell the difference between being hurt & being injured. I am hurt, as anyone with this large of a mass that suddenly starts to expect their body to do more than it has in the past couple decades would be, but I am not injured. I look at it like this: injured means I need medical attention. Hurt, on the other hand, means I can choose to push through some pain to try to reach my goal, or I can tuck my tail & assume the fetal position till the bit of discomfort goes away. Needless to say, I went with walking through the pain. I even added another half a mile to my route; I figured if I am going to push through the pain I might as well make it as hard of a push as possible. I walk the same route every time (of course with another half mile lap added today), so I see the same people over & over. At first I have to admit I was a bit cautious, figuring people in much better shape than me would be laughing at the fat cow as he sweat & struggled through a little walk. But I would say the opposite is true. The people I know in my neighborhood who are fellow fatties are the ones who act like, "What do you think you are doing?" Those in good shape, however, those who clearly take care of themselves, offer kind waves & words of encouragement. I have a theory about this: some of your fellow fatties don't want you bettering yourself, because they will have to take a look at themselves, which is why some of your fat friends may react less than kindly to your efforts. On the other hand, those who do make the effort to take care of themselves know how hard it is to motivate to work out, so when they see you do it they know you are struggling with a lot more than they are, yet you are still out there.

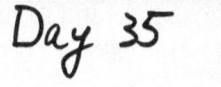

Sunday, & we headed to a fine southern gun show. My wife couldn't make it; she's out of commission with a summer stomach flu. The gun show was good, but why do they have to have a concession stand there? Seriously I could have done without watching people pound hamburgers & cheese fries down their throats! I wanted to be one of those people! I managed to resist the cheeseburger & cheese fries value meal; luckily I had a bar with me—yeah that was just as good. So mental note: be prepared for temptation to challenge you anywhere & everywhere. It's bad enough that my church will often offer doughnuts Sunday morning, but hey I know to expect that. There are times when all you can do to get through unexpected temptation is to suck it up & tell yourself you are stronger than your cravings.

Day 36
Weight: 274.6
Loss week 5: 4 pounds
Loss to date: 33.8 pounds

Sub 275! Needless to say, I am a happy camper. At this weight I am wearing a size 40 pants; if I hit my goal I should be buying pants in the 30s for the first time in a very long time. Oh yeah! I can buy regular clothes. I won't have to count the Xs in front of the large or head to the end of the rack & hope the pants come in at a big enough size. A friend said he could really tell that I have lost weight, & I know he wasn't just blowing smoke. Hell, I am ninety percent of the man I was thirty-six days ago! As an added bonus this week I get to move the fattest clothes I have out of my closet! No more of those triple-X shirts & size 44 pants taking up space. So I made it through another day: bars, shakes, & chicken, romaine lettuce & cucumber. I am amazed I haven't wavered at all from this program. A couple other people I know who have been on this program cheated within the first two weeks, & a couple others modified it from the start. Somehow (I am going to say it's pure desperation to be less fat) I have managed to stay the course for the first thirty-six days.

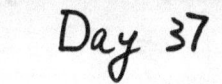

Day 37

Movie day. If it seems like a common occurrence that's because it is. I usually go to the movies once a week. I used to look forward to the candy but I can tell you it doesn't make the movie any more enjoyable—to be frank, it's nice to save the few bucks by bringing a bar. The tough part is that our local movie theater sells pizza. Yep, pizza at the movies! Mind you, not good pizza, but to me even bad pizza is better than most things. However, I managed to resist. I am up to forty minutes of walking at this point & will increase that another ten minutes next week.

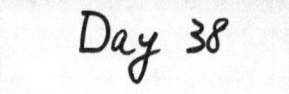

Day 38

Spent about three hours working on the lawn, another part of my regular workout routine since it seems like I am doing it every week. Amazing how much easier it is to do basic things like yard work. At 300-plus everything was just so damn difficult. Everyone keeps saying how much weight I've lost & how good I look, but I still see a fat man in the mirror. Obviously I am still fat: I am over 270, & that's fat, no way around it—but for now, at least, I am less fat & that is progress. All in all, another rather easy day to stay with the program. Hey, two easy days in a row: maybe I have turned the corner & the days of painful temptation are over? Somehow I don't think so.

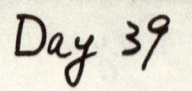

Day 39

Snuck on the scale again today: 272. I am still waiting for the first pla-teau to hit but hopefully I can keep one step ahead of it. Today wasn't as easy of a day to resist food temptations. I had to go to the grocery since my wife is sick. Let me tell you, the people who put together grocery stores are pure evil! I started getting some chicken & had to clear the pastries, cupcakes, & fresh-made cookies & bread. Then I went to get a couple cans of soup for my wife—for some reason, the soup aisle is also the candy aisle! How are soup & candy in any way related? Then I went to get some cotton swabs &, what do I find but cookies sitting right next to them. Last is the soda & of course you have chips of all sorts in that aisle. I don't really know my way around the grocery (not one of my normal chores), so I had to keep walking around facing endless temptations. Then its check out time. As I wait somewhat patiently, the lady in front of me decides, after she has been rung up, that she needs a chocolate bar the evil bastards put right in front of you as you wait to leave. She actually said, "I need that. It's been one of those days." Wow, do I know what she means.

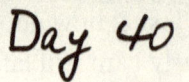

Day 40

Went through the closet; time to move those fat clothes the hell out of there! I can tell you every pair of pants bigger than a size 40 was way too big. Also, for the first time in a long time, I am wearing my pants at my actual waist & not under the gut. I have fewer clothing options but I couldn't be happier! Based on this progress, another twenty pounds & I will be buying size 38 pants.

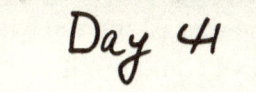

I woke up last night in unbearable pain. I could barely stand as I tried to walk off the aching in my right hamstring. As I tried to walk it off the front of my knee starting sending me a pulsing pain message. This was about four hours after I had gone to bed. It took me a good hour before the leg wasn't killing me. I spent the entire day a little out of it from the lack of sleep & the startling wake up. Went to look at a weight bench, picked up new walking sneakers (in the hopes that the old, beat-up sneakers I was wearing might be part of the problem), & did my forty minutes of walking. If you want basic walking sneakers without paying for the fancy ad campaign you can get them for around forty bucks. If they work & I don't wake up in that kind of pain anytime soon, then it might be the best forty bucks I ever made. I really need to keep a better eye on the shape of my sneakers & not be so cheap & replace them when they need to be replaced. I am happy to have made it through a tough, pain-filled day without breaking & sticking to the walking. If I can make it through a day like today, then there is a good chance I should be able to make it through any day.

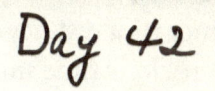

Got a weight bench today, spent a whole hundred bucks on it. After seeing the host of options, most in the $250-plus range, I decided on a simple bench for my simple workout. Seriously, the equipment means very little; it's what you do with it that counts. We had a long conversation with our neighbor tonight regarding her weight. She is twenty-five & obese & she was asking me what I did & how I managed to do it. The best way I could put it was that you have to undo a lifetime worth of mental training & re-educate your brain to think differently about food. For me, I know it's thirty-seven years worth of mental training that I have been fighting. Intellectually I have always known the endless pizza, cookies, ice cream, & candy weren't good for me. So it's not an intellectual fight; it's deeper than that. It's deep-seated, subconscious training you are trying to overcome, & that takes a lot of hard work & determination to beat.

Day 43
Weight: 268.8

Loss week 6: 5.8 pounds

Loss to date: 39.7 pounds

I never thought I would be in the 260s this early. I was shocked. So shocked I had to get on the scale twice & have my wife come over to make sure I was reading the number right. Just flat out awesome. I can't believe I have lost forty pounds in forty-three days! When you think about it, I lost a toddler! Today is the first day I am doing weights, which is good since it's a rest day from walking so my knee doesn't explode. It has been a long time since I have even picked up a weight so the pounds I was pushing were pathetic—so pathetic that I can't bring myself to type them. Much like starting the diet, this is going to be a process that I will have to get used to. I kept the weight training simple: two exercises for the chest, two for the back, two for the triceps, & two for the biceps. We booked the California trip. We will be out there for six days. Normally on a vacation I eat myself sick & then buy bigger pants. But I am dedicated to making this trip a net neutral. I figure if I can deal with a wedding & reception, a trip to my sister's (did I mention my sister is a really good cook?), enjoy good-tasting but bad for me foods with friends I haven't seen in almost a year, & come back not having gained any weight it will be a success. So far the plan looks like this: we booked a hotel with a gym in it & a refrigerator so I can buy the precooked grilled chicken I like. Then we decided we would walk the beach near our old house a couple times (that's a good 3.5 miles with hills), and I am bringing thirty bars with me.

Day 44

Wow, was I sore today. If it's been a while since you have picked up a weight, prepare for it to suck the next day. All my joints are screaming at me. I guess when you go so long without picking up anything heavier than an extra-large pizza box, you should expect pain. Today was a light day, just walking. I feel like I am in some weird limbo: on one hand I know I have lost a good amount of weight & can see it in the way my clothes fit; on the other hand I am still really fat. Today was one of those days when I simply did not want to be on a diet. I did stick to it, but it was a tough day. I don't know if it has something to do with wanting to reward myself or not, but I can tell you my traditional reward for a job well done has been food. I had that "I deserve a pizza" thought hit me often today. So even after forty pounds & over forty days, I am here to say you will still be fighting that fat piggy that lives deep inside you.

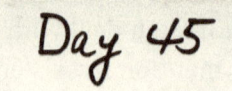

Okay today I pushed it: weights & walking. I know it doesn't sound like much to some but for me, or anyone in my shape, it might as well be the Iron Man. On top of that, today was one of those hot & muggy southern days, one of those days that just drains you. Even my wife, my biggest supporter in this massive effort to be less massive, was offering amnesty from my walk. What makes the difference on the scale, though, is doing it when you really, really don't want to, when you have every reason not to: you're hurt, you're tired, it's too hot, blah, blah, blah. That's when you have to suck it up & do it if you want results.

Day 46

As is typical I snuck on the scale today: 264.8! I am officially sub 265! Next stop, 250s! I guess forty-five days of bars, grilled chicken, romaine lettuce, & cucumbers has paid off. That's what gastro bypass patients see & they risk their lives in surgery & have their stomachs cut to the size of a tablespoon. Add this to the long list of pluses to losing weight: I used to need a good two hours to get out of the house in the morning, slowly dragging my fat butt into the waking world. Well, this morning I was able to get up, have coffee, feed & walk the dog, weigh myself, shower, shave, get dressed, & get out of the house in under an hour. Amazingly, the joints were a lot less sore from working out today. I no longer seem to need the knee brace for my walks. Today I had a great pace going; I was close to jogging! I want to add another half a mile, which will take me to a little over 3 miles next week, then add another half mile a week the following two weeks & then I will try jogging some of it. I went to the grocery store today: the usual chicken, lettuce, cucumbers, and I also got myself a couple men's fitness magazines. Yeah, I know, no big deal, right? Well, this is the first time I have ever bought these types of magazines without suffering shame. I am actually starting to look like someone who cares about his health and, more importantly, seeing myself as someone who cares about his health.

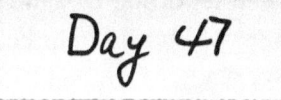

Day 47

Today my wife went for pizza and I had a bar & the joy of trying not to kill myself lifting weights. Who said life is fair, right? Not that I would break at this point for pizza; I mean, I can see myself in the 240s in the next thirty days & change. I wouldn't risk that success for anything at this point. I never thought I would still have a noticeable fat roll after losing forty-five pounds. Next week I should clear the fifty-pound mark: that's half a hundred & still there will be fat hanging out. Sure, I have lost a lot & it's noticeable: my size 40 pants are too big, which tells me I would be buying size 38 pants at this point. Also, a lot of the 2x T-shirts are tents on me—but the fat roll persists.

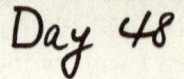

Today is a great example of why I only do weights every other day: sore is an understatement. The odd thing is I am not pushing a lot of weight at all, but my shoulder is killing me. There is some past damage there, so I try to be as careful as possible. The walk is getting too easy; Monday I will be adding another six tenths of a mile, which will take me to around 3.2 miles. I will keep adding a lap around my neighborhood (one lap is six tenths of a mile) a week for the next four weeks, that way I will be doing five miles of walking six days a week. That gradual increase should help keep the plateaus at bay. Sleep is still an issue; I have a hard time getting to bed before three; I simply am not tired. Someday I have to figure this out because I have read that lack of sleep can seriously reduce weight loss.

Day 49

It's official: I made it seven weeks. Okay, I know this diet seems severe & extreme but I have never been a successful dieter & I have managed to stay on it for seven weeks so clearly it isn't impossible to stick to. The combination of my desperation because of health issues and the huge successes I have had week after week make it possible for me to stick with it. I have lived forty-nine days on less than 1000 calories a day and I survived! Researching restaurant food for my trip I can tell you it's tough to leave any restaurant & not consume 1500 calories in one meal. However, I will be attempting to keep all my meals, even though I am on vacation, within the 500-range. By cutting bread—having an open-face sandwich or a hamburger with lettuce as the bun—ordering beans or salad instead of French fries as a side dish, & not having appetizers or desserts I ought to be able to do it. Another thing to keep in mind for my vacation food adventures is portion control. Restaurants love to stack your plate beyond what anyone should eat. I like the fist-size rule. I know if I eat more than that then I overate; it is an easy way to keep track of you intake.

> ## Day 50
> Weight: 262.8
>
> Loss week 7: 6 pounds
>
> Loss to date: 45.7 pounds

Looking back, I think the weight training I added last week is what kept the loss going at such a good rate. I am 4.3 pounds shy of hitting the 50-pound loss mark: that's like half a super model! Living on less than a thousand calories a day does not provide a lot of fuel for working out. The walking is doable, but when you add weight training you can't expect your body to magically produce fuel. Today I was able to increase the walking by six-tenths of a mile, so I am now walking 3.2 miles six days a week. I walked by a couple neighbors who joked that I walk too fast—a nice compliment I never thought I'd hear. I try to keep the pace up so I am basically panting all the way through the walk. That way I am getting the best cardio I can without having to step up to a jog.

Day 51

I have been doing some reading & from what I've found, six hours or less of sleep a night actually leads to weight gain, while seven to eight hours a night promotes weight loss. I knew weight loss & sleep were tied together but I didn't know to what degree. I found a great article about how restaurants use what I dubbed the "death triangle" in preparing their goods: salt, fat, & sugar. Oddly enough this combo gives us the greatest satisfaction from food & gets us to keep coming back regardless how bad the food is for us. Think about French fries: now I love French fries, but they are typically deep fried in fat before they are packaged & then deep fried again when you order them, then covered in salt & served with ketchup, which is full of sugar. Even something that seems harmless, like the chips they bring you at a Mexican restaurant, aren't so harmless. The chips are deep fried, salted, & then served with salsa, which contains sugar. I knew about the 1500-calorie salads & 2400-calorie burger meals but come on, how can someone watch their weight & ever eat out? My advice: be careful eating out, research where you are eating prior to going so you know what you are going to order before you show up, feel free to order off the menu or change a dish if you need to, and avoid the weight inflating free offerings they bring to the table.

Day 52

So far I have lost close to fifty pounds, but when I look in the mirror I still see a fat guy. I had to ask my wife how much fatter I was fifty pounds ago? More importantly, why didn't anyone say anything? See

I always assumed I was about fifty pounds overweight & if I was able to lose that weight I would look great. Well not so. Not that I don't look a lot better; I do. However, there is still clearly a lot more work to do. So she told me she couldn't say anything, & it wasn't really her place to, that she loved me no matter what. That is a problem us fatties are going to have to deal with: those who love us usually won't let us know we might want to put down the cookies & pick up a barbell. Of course, it's easy to see her point of view: who would want to tell their spouse they are getting way too fat? Friends & other family are in the same situation; it's just not right for them to confront us fatties. So we are left having to be honest with ourselves.

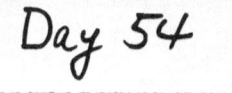

Day 53

It is amazing how much easier this is getting. I am actually used to the walking & the diet & slowly getting use to the weight training. After fifty-plus days, the diet seems like a regular routine, as if eating something else would be weird. Of course I plan on testing that theory once I am on my vacation next week.

Day 54

Got on the scale this morning: 257.8! I am in the 250s for the first time in a long time! Seeing that number really made all the work & dieting worth it. Today's walk was really easy; I kept repeating 255, 255, 255; over & over again. That's the next number I want to see & I want to see it ASAP. Even on a hot & muggy southern evening I kept a great pace. Nothing is as motivating as results. Not only has my metabolism changed, the highly structured diet has given me the chance to reset my thoughts about food. Perfect example: today I was talking to my wife about our upcoming vacation. She has a favorite sandwich shop, & I told her I could go with her, but instead of ordering what I would have before, the large meatball parmesan, I am going to order the regular turkey with mustard, cheese, & red onion. What I want is a sandwich & in reality any sandwich is going to bring me the same degree of satisfaction, so why not go with the healthier option?

Day 55

Today was one tough day. It was muggy, 100 degrees, & I was totally out of gas. The only thing I managed to do was sleep on the couch & go to the grocery store. I was supposed to do weights today, but there was no chance in hell I could. My body was just completely gassed. These days are going to hit me from time to time, since I have so few calories to work with & am doing both weights & cardio. Anyway, there comes a point when we all have to listen to our bodies, & for me that day was today.

Day 56

Okay the day of rest yesterday was worth it; even though it was as hot & muggy today I felt one hundred percent better. Even got my 3.2 miles of cardio in. I did sneak back on the scale: my weight was exactly the same, 257.8, so yesterday didn't cost me anything I guess. Tomorrow I am hoping to see a number in the 256–range; maybe wishful thinking, but one can dream.

Day 57
Weight: 256.6

Loss week 8: 6.2 pounds

Loss to date: 51.8 pounds

Chest: 45, loss to date, 2 inches

Waist: 40.5, loss to date, 6 inches

Abs: 43.75, loss to date; 5.25 inches

Arms; 13.5, loss to date, 1 inch

Thigh: 25.5, loss to date, 1.75 inch

Well hoping & praying actually works. I don't know how much longer the six pounds a week loss will keep up but I plan to enjoy that ride as long as I can. The inches lost is pretty impressive as well, based on everything I have read. Today was a really active day, did weights, three hours of yard work, & walked. I didn't add the six-tenths of a mile to the walk yet; figured I can wait until tomorrow to do that since I was already almost dead on my feet by the time I hit the road.

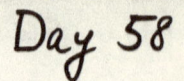

While discussing weight loss with a fellow fatty, we came up with a new weight range: doughy. Doughy, our new goal, is someone who is maybe twenty pounds or less overweight, but works out; basically someone who looks like they know where both the gym & the best pizza places are. What we have to keep in mind is our wants & goals, not some ideal of perfection. The media has gone out of its way to poison our heads. You hear all the talk about women's body image issues, but what about us guys? Unrealistic expectations are thrown our way all the time as well. A lot of guys toil through their lives killing themselves to get to an ideal at the expense of every other aspect of their life. I would rather be healthy & look good & be able to go to a pizza parlor with my family than have to do double cardio days & spend three hours away from my family at the gym to strive for an ideal. My wife is on the same page: she wants me healthy so I can enjoy my life & live longer but she really doesn't care if I have an eight-pack or not. She actually thinks I look damn good now. Women can be easy to please, thank God.

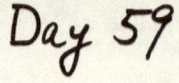

Just weights today. Since I have a structured program in place I might as well share it at this point. I do feel obligated to add the caveat that I am not an exercise expert; the following was based on my own research. My suggestion is do your own homework & come up with a program that you believe in & that you will actually do, which is much more important that figuring out the "perfect" program. I do two exercises for each body part & do the whole routine every other day:

Chest: bench press, inclined bench press

Upper back: shrugs, back rows

Biceps: barbell curls, hammer curls

Triceps: triceps extension, French press

Abs: leg lifts, dumbbell obliques

I got to this program by trial & error; because of past injuries I moved things in & out of the routine based on what didn't strain an existing injury. You have to make it something you can do without hurting yourself. The purpose isn't to hurt yourself; it is to build muscle, which you have to do that over time. If you hurt yourself you won't be able to do the next workout. Now I won't share the weight amounts I use, because I still have a little pride left, but I will tell you I use weights that I can do three sets of ten reps that push my muscles without causing any serious pain. I don't do any leg exercises because my cardio is walking & I do have bad knees. I don't want to risk hurting something that would make me skip the cardio. The best part is that all of this is done using a basic weight bench & some basic weights, so there's no big cost & no need for a monthly gym membership. Not that there is anything wrong with a gym membership, but the point is that this can be done with very little cost. We might have spent one hundred dollars on the weights & another one hundred on a basic bench. All of the cardio of course is free; all I had to do was buy a forty-dollar pair of sneakers. So, for less than $250 bucks, I have an exercise program that has helped me shed over fifty pounds: not a bad ROI.

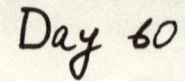

Day 60

Sixty days on this diet is amazing for someone who has never successfully dieted. Of course, losing fifty-five pounds in those sixty days makes sticking with it a lot easier. I have been stuck at the same weight the last couple days. Yeah, I am hitting the scale daily at this point, but hey, I have a limited amount of time left. Don't know why the scale isn't moving; to be honest I have no idea what to change to make it start moving down again. I can't really cut calories since there are none to cut & it's not like I can increase my exercise, since, as I said, there are no calories so I am running on no fuel as it is. Hopefully the next couple days prove fruitful & the scale starts moving in the right direction soon.

Day 61

Scale moved about a pound today, which is better than nothing. I was hoping to be under 250 by Monday, but that most likely won't happen. It is getting harder & harder to stick with the program as I increase my exercising & feel more & more gassed as the days go on. It is tough when the results come slowly; it was a lot easier to keep on it when I was shedding a couple pounds every couple days. What keeps me on it now is the fact that I have a break coming up for my vacation in a couple weeks. I promised myself I would enjoy my vacation, within reason, so all I need to do is keep on the program until then.

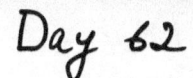

Day 62

Today was a tough day, a day where I basically did nothing. Temperature was in the high 90s & the humidity was high, so I sat & sweated through this Saturday. I had planned on walking but a huge rainstorm hit, so my walk was cancelled. This is a good reason to have indoor cardio equipment, because the weather doesn't always agree with your workout plans. Hopefully tomorrow is a better day.

Day 63

Okay, today was an AWESOME day. Since it was stinking hot again I took the wife to the mall, figuring since my closet is all but empty I might want to pick up a few things. I am not a huge shopping fan, but this was fun. My clothes were all at least two sizes smaller, & my suit size dropped three sizes! I was shocked. It is amazing what a difference fifty pounds can make. So, as you probably guessed, once we got back from the mall I did weights & my four-plus miles of walking that night—and did it with a big dumb grin.

Day 64
Weight: 251.4
Loss week 9: 5.2 pounds
Loss to date: 57 pounds

I met a business associate for a meeting today, dressed in my new smaller clothes, & the first words out of his mouth were, "You look like a completely different person." That was good to hear. The last time he saw me I was twenty pounds heavier, so I guess even twenty pounds makes a difference. When I look at old three-hundred-pound-plus pictures I really do look like a different person. Even my face is smaller. So after the kind words & good day I pounded through my four-mile walk hoping to see continued results.

Day 65

Sixty-five straight days of eating the exact same things without any variations. Talk about extreme: even inmates get a little variety. I am looking forward to my week vacation; I am going to allow myself to eat a bit more freely, and, hopefully, I can recharge my determination so I can come back to battle the rest of my bulge. My knee & both my hips are killing me. I may be overdoing the exercise a bit. I will stick with it for now & suffer through, until I get to my vacation goal.

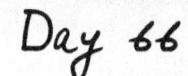

Day 66

Ah, another benefit of shedding that excess weight: my wife can't keep her hands off me. She is so shocked by how different I look after dropping sixty pounds. I can't say I blame her; I do look a lot better. Today I was buried in work so the exercise was minimal; hopefully there will be no ill effects on the scale.

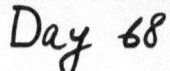

Day 67

Picked up my new suits from the tailor today. If you manage to shed fifty pounds, go get a new suit. You will look a thousand times better than you ever have in a suit. I cut the walk by about half a mile today. It is much more important to be able to walk six days a week then it is to walk farther on fewer days—at least that's my theory. I hit another achievement today: 247.8! I am officially sixty pounds lighter & under 250 pounds for the first time in over two decades!

Day 68

I got a good workout on the weights today; I was able to increase the weight amount for every exercise, so I am making progress. Tomorrow is the July 4, a great eating holiday. I will be hiding out in the house. Of course burgers, fries, corn on the cob, ice cream, cookies, cakes, etc., all sound good, but I have only a few days left to keep on the program before my vacation & I am determined to do so. I went to the grocery today—bad idea. It was pre-Fourth of July shopping day & the carts were packed full of crap nobody should eat but that I would love to.

Day 69

Ah, the Fourth of July: no barbeque for me this year, no sweet treats. Maybe next year if I am in good enough shape I can host a healthier Fourth of July party. That's one of my goals: to show others ways to easily cut calories while still enjoying what you eat so that gaining weight is no longer a problem. Of course first I will have to figure that out for myself since I don't think a bar and shake party would get a lot of positive RSVPs. The scale went up a pound today, which was to be expected even though I did cardio & weights yesterday. Yeah, the scale will do that, which is why you shouldn't weigh yourself every day. I don't see 238.5 being realistic, but if I can get under 242 then I will have the three pounds of wiggle room I wanted so that if my vacation adds two to three pounds in a week I am still at a good weight & can get back on track when we get back.

Day 70

"You no longer look like a rock. Did your wife put you in the dryer?" That's what I heard from someone I haven't seen since I went on this diet. I guess dropping sixty pounds, twenty percent of your old body weight, makes an impact. I must say I was more than motivated to pump the weights today; I was able to increase the weight amounts on most exercises. Again, nothing impressive, but still an improvement, which is what I am always looking for. You can't get caught up in how much weight you're moving; instead, focus on how much more weight you are moving than you did before. Hopefully tomorrow I see something in the 245-range, but no matter what I am already in the best shape of my life & loving every moment of it.

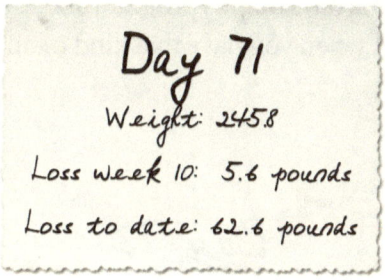

Day 71

Weight: 245.8

Loss week 10: 5.6 pounds

Loss to date: 62.6 pounds

That was a pleasant surprise! Now I am starting to think, *Hey, maybe I can get under 240 before the wedding.* Got to love the mind games weight loss does to you. I was thinking of how we make such deep-seated, emotional, subconscious connections to food. Classic example: a parent rewards a child for doing well in school with food. That child gets enough of that in their head then, as an adult, they feel success should be rewarded with food (as I always did). The same goes for the parent who comforts their kids with ice cream. What is that child going to want when they have a rough day as an adult? I struggle with this, as do most of us. Every day for the past seventy-one days I have gone twelve rounds with my own subconscious. The good thing is you can make new connections in your subconscious, as I have been doing. I am slowly training my subconscious to see food differently. I really believe that is essential for long-term success. That's the goal: not just to shed some weight that comes back on, but to lose it and keep it off for life.

Day 72

Great day today: weighed in at 244! Don't know what it was. I tried to stay really active yesterday, so maybe that helped. Ran around all day & then did cardio. Some days on this program are just awesome; it makes it easier to stick to it when you have that kind of one-day success.

Day 73

Damn scale. Seriously, damn scale. Damn thing tells me 245.2 this morning! Maybe it's broken—or better yet, maybe I should break it. That was my morning—& you thought yours sucked. The southern summer weather didn't cooperate with my planned walk tonight. It's really hard to walk when it is pouring down rain for four hours. I spent my planned cardio time researching supplements. Wow, is there a lot of information out there. Supplements can be dangerous territory; some are pure garbage, & some are downright danger-ous. I am keeping it simple: a low calorie protein shake and cre-atine to help with recovery. Creatine naturally occurs in your body. Those who weight train benefit from taking it by decreasing needed recovery time & reducing fatigue while increasing muscle size & strength. My plan is to give them both a month once I get back from vacation & see how well they work.

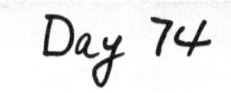

Day 74

Today the scale moved back down to 243.4. Talk about relieved. My morning started a lot better than yesterday. I did weights today as well as cardio. As usual, success on the scale brings newfound energy to make it through workouts.

Day 75

Scale stayed at 243.4 today. I am fine with that, considering I got hit with a massive sinus infection. Got to love getting sick when you are trying to get something done. Needless to say I did zero exercise today, since breathing is sort of important to the workout process & not something I can do well right now. As important as reaching my goals is the fact that I won't get anywhere if I don't listen to my body. Today my body told me to get a couple of movies & park my butt on the couch.

Day 76

Today's good news: the scale went down to 242.2. The bad news: my company's website went haywire today, so after spending most of the day in programming hell my wife talked me into ordering a pizza. I know: seventy-five days of strict dieting and today I have a pizza. Well, she also wanted to see if I was going to get sick to my stomach from regular food before we are in California. We both would rather me get sick here than there. So we ordered a light pizza: thin crust, light sauce, light cheese, & onion. Although I didn't get that "full and happy belly" effect from pizza like I used to, I did enjoy it and my stomach was fine. I figure I had about seven hundred calories so hopefully I don't see any increase in the scale tomorrow. I still couldn't exercise today; still not feeling good at all. Hopefully I'll feel better tomorrow & can get back to working out.

Day 77

The scale was exactly the same as yesterday: 242.2. I guess I can safely eat light pizza without risking gaining any weight, right? Well, maybe not on a nightly basis, but on occasion, maybe. I felt good all day; I think the pizza break really helped. I did weights & cardio today, getting a really good workout in. In three days we leave on vacation & I can't wait. We need a break, & I know I need a break from this program for a few days.

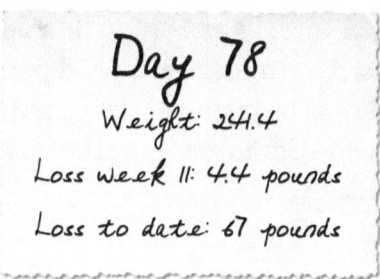

Day 78

Weight: 244.4

Loss week 11: 4.4 pounds

Loss to date: 67 pounds

A nice little drop today. Of course I most likely won't be under 240 by Wednesday but I really shouldn't complain; dropping sixty-seven pounds in seventy-eight days is nothing to shake a stick at. I need to start doing weights on one day & cardio the next; this beat-up body can't handle doing both on the same day at this point. I was wrecked today. I really didn't do much but pack & wrap up a few work items so I can vacation in peace.

Day 79

I have no explanation for this one: 239.8 today. I did neither cardio nor weights yesterday & I only got about four hours of sleep. I only did a little yard work, some general work around the house, & packed. Some days the scale is just unexplainable. Today is our last day before we fly to California. In honor of our upcoming vacation, we ordered a pizza. Why not, since I am under 240? Of course we had thin crust, light sauce, light cheese, and onions, and tonight we added grilled chicken. I would say it was much better & much more filling with the grilled chicken on it. Today I skipped the weights & cardio; I don't want to be all banged up & hurting when I fly tomorrow. Our hotel gym only has cardio equipment so we are bringing some of those workout bands my wife has. I have never used them before: another adventure. I just want to be able to keep some sort of program together & of course get a good pump before the wedding. There are going to be pictures taken and I might as well look as good as I can, right? Got to get some decent sleep tonight, since tomorrow is travel day.

Day 80

Flight day. Air travel is not exactly the perfect environment for a dieter. Our six hours of air travel turned into a fifteen-hour affair that included a missed flight, a nice run through an airport that proved fruitless, & a conversation with TSA officials. Needless to say, a ton of stress for one day. The airports *do* offer a lot of comfort food to ease your travel pains. I packed a handful of bars in my carry-on so I was able to stay with the program. After our fifteen-hour travel adventure we ordered pizza—again the harmless variety, light sauce & cheese, thin crust, & grilled chicken. I checked out the "workout center" at the hotel; that phrase is a huge overestimation. A couple of beat-up treadmills & bikes don't make a workout center. It's pretty pathetic actually. We plan on walking the beach; might as well suck up some of the finer Southern California offerings. If you are traveling, plan on the hotel's gym offering to be minimal. They did put a small refrigerator in the room, so at least we can keep food & water so we won't have an endless array of take-out & sit-down fattening feasts. Tonight a family we knew came by the room—what a look of shock. She hadn't seen me since I was over three hundred pounds so she was a bit floored.

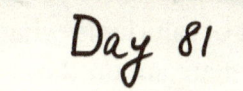

Day 81

I felt great this morning & no bigger from my pizza indulgence. We went & picked up some food for the room and I went with bars until dinner. Dinner tonight was with two very good friends of mine who were shocked to see the change. One has known me for almost two decades & he couldn't believe it. Even though they knew how much I had lost, the number of pounds don't translate as well as the visual. My wife took a picture of us & I can see my success in it. I still see myself as a fat guy who has thirty more pounds to drop but the progress I have made is clear in pictures. We went to Mexican restaurant & I tried to keep on the program by ordering chicken fajitas, but they season & sauce them so much I know there were a lot more calories than I am used to. The chicken serving was actually small; I would say maybe four ounces & I am used to six. If you don't use all the fattening unhealthy crap they bring you to put on the fajitas you don't get much of a meal. Our dinner conversation was interesting; we focused solely on my weight-loss success. It was odd being asked weight loss advice, I never thought I would be the person to dole out advice on that subject! I actually felt a bit off after dinner; I could tell it wasn't the clean food I have become used to.

Day 82

I woke up feeling okay. I had a bar & coffee for breakfast, then lunch with an old friend at a famous wings place. We used to eat lunch there every Friday for a couple years so it was more about tradition than food. I only had a few wings, trying to keep the damage to a minimum. There are a lot of calories in wings, especially when you consider how little meat there are on those bones. We walked the beach today, as I haven't exercised since we got here & am starting to feel it. We used to do this walk on occasion when we lived here & it would almost kill me. What a wonder dropping almost seventy pounds can make. Dinner didn't go as planned; by the time we got back everything was closed so I had to go with a room service burger. After not having beef in the past eighty-two days it was really hard to digest. I felt like I was nine months pregnant for hours & couldn't wait for the baby to bust out.

Day 83

Today's was the wedding. I did almost nothing most of the day as my wife ran around getting her hair & make-up done, as I enjoyed my bars. The wedding was awesome. People I haven't seen in seventy pounds were absolutely shocked. Someone even guessed I weighed two hundred pounds—seriously, two hundred pounds!—and nobody could see how I could want to drop another thirty pounds although I can easily see where that thirty pounds would come from. When I told people what I had done to lose the weight, I heard a dozen times from people looking to drop some pounds that they could never do that. I assure you that if I can than anyone can. I kept my reception eating in check: a small serving of pasta, a couple rolls, a large salad, and, of course, a small piece of cake.

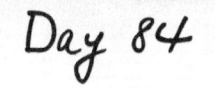

Day 84

I went down to my see my sister & mom today & let me tell you, their shock was awesome. My mom actually felt bad for me since I don't enjoy eating anymore. She wanted to feed me so badly it was actually kind of funny. I wonder where my reliance on food for comfort comes from! My sister has put on some weight recently and asked me what I did to lose weight. When I told her and showed her a bar (I ate bars for everything but dinner, even as they kept offering me food), she said there was no way she could do that. Dinner was rough; my sister made a great barbeque chicken. It was the best thing I have eaten this entire trip & inspired me to buy a barbeque when I get home. My mom made her special potato salad, which I have always loved, but since it probably has 1000 calories per forkful I tried not to eat too much of it, but it was so good. The rough part was the ice cream cake for my niece's birthday. When I told them I wanted to lose another thirty pounds she said if I lost any more weight I would look gaunt. Talk about funny—gaunt, really. It can be tough for family to see you in a new light, especially when the change is so drastic & affects not only the way you look but also the way you live. Pretty soon they will see me as I am living now & this will become as normal to them as it is becoming to me.

Day 85

Last day of vacation & I spent most of it helping the newlyweds move. I guess my new fit look makes me a better invite to last-minute moving parties. I got a good workout in, hauling crap up &

down the stairs. We went to dinner at a Mexican place with some friends & I had chicken tacos. They were pretty good, just grilled chicken & cilantro. In California, by law restaurants have to provide the nutritional information of their menu, an idea that should become law nationwide. I like knowing what I am going to put in my body. That information actually made me change my selection. I am so ready to get back home, back to my normal eating & exercise routine and curious to see what the scale has to say.

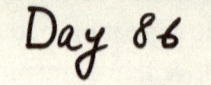

Flight day. Again, not the ideal situation to stick with any sort of diet program. I kept to the bars most of the day; the only break was cheese crackers at one of the three airports in which I had the joy of spending time. A woman who sat next to me on one flight woofed down a fast-food salad; she could have just ordered a burger and fries because a dressing-drenched salad with fried chicken on top isn't any better for you. Got home, unpacked, piled up a stack of clothes to be washed, ate a bag of popcorn, & went to bed. Really don't want to see what that scale says tomorrow.

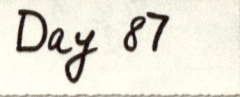

243.3: I gained 3.3 pounds in 7 days. Amazing what wandering off the path will do, isn't it? One of the big mistakes I made is not drinking enough water, so today I drank a ton of water, since over vacation I was pounding diet sodas. Another little slip I failed to mention is eating crackers at night. My wife bought a box of crackers & I figured why not, I am on vacation—bad idea. We ordered pizza tonight, again the same light cheese & sauce, thin crust, chicken, & onion we have been ordering. I figured, why not? It is my first day of post-vacation recovery right? I will need a couple days to get back into the swing of things; I figure by Monday I will be back on track & by the following Monday I will be back under 240.

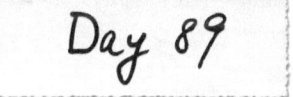

Day 88

It's the second day home & to be honest I am having a hard time getting back on track. I have not done one bit of exercise yet. At least I didn't order pizza tonight, so there is a start. Maybe I need a couple more days to get myself back on the program. I guess time will tell.

Day 89

Okay down to 242.8 today. At least the scale is moving in the right direction again. I did some yard work today; again no actual exercise but better than nothing. Ordered a pizza again. Did I mention I am having a hard time getting back on the program? I also have introduced salt-free peanuts into my diet. I seem to be addicted to them at this point; can't shake the peanut cravings. Not that it is a bad thing, all things considered, but still not really part of the program. We will see what the impact is on the scale.

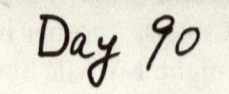

240! Oh yeah. Guess pizza & peanuts aren't so bad for you? I did drink a lot of water yesterday & I also did that yard work. Getting back on track is harder than it was to get going the first time around! I just can't work up the motivation. At this point I can no longer claim it's jetlag; clearly the lazy part of my brain has taken over again. So again we ordered pizza, figured since I am 240 why not.

Day 91

Still no exercise. Still can't find the proper motivation. Hell, I can't find *any* motivation.

Day 92

Wow: 239 today; the pizza diet is working. No exercise today but we had water ice, my wife's idea. She figured I deserved a treat before going back on the program. The thing you read about sugar making you crave more sugar is one hundred percent true: the birthday cake-flavored water ice made the rest of the day a lot harder as I kept chasing a sugar craving. Next time I am going to go with the sugar-free variety. Oh & of course I had the large—if you are going to screw up, screw up big.

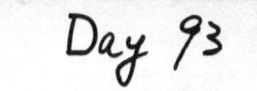

Damn, 241 today. I guess we now know how bad a large sugar–filled, birthday cake-flavored water ice can be. Two things I know for sure: I am not ordering any more pizza, & I have to start exercising in the hopes of bringing that scale back down.

Day 94

Finally got some exercise in: a 3.5-mile walk, which is a start. My feet are killing me; expected when you sit on your butt for a couple weeks & your feet don't get used. I really don't look forward to hitting the weights again; I can only imagine the pain I am in for. Seriously, when you get yourself on a workout program, stay on it no matter what! Don't make the stupid mistake I did. I stayed off the scale today for my mental health; it is amazing how one pound the wrong way can ruin your day. Monday I hope to see something in the 237-range. May be wishful thinking but one can hope, right? Hoping paid off in the early part of the program; maybe hope is ready for an encore. If I see a decent number I will leave the peanuts in the diet, if not then they go away & it is back to following the diet strictly.

CHAPTER THREE
AN UNPLANNED HIATUS

I am going off the program for a bit. Come on, did you really think I was going to keep at this pace? Seriously? Did you skip the part where I said I was undoing thirty-seven years worth of training? Did you expect that to be easy?

I need a break from this program at this point. Reversing thirty-seven years of training isn't easy, clearly. This hiatus is a bit unplanned; I figured at some point I would need it, but the timing is completely unplanned. It's just a series of events that led me here; I know this is the right time to take it.

So how did I spend the hiatus? Well, you know how they say old habits are hard to break? They weren't lying to you. In some respects I fell right back into my old routine: spending a lot of time sitting on my butt & ignoring both weight training & cardio. You have to have sympathy for my couch. The hardest thing about long-formed habits is figuring out how to break them. We can't help but go back to our comfort zones, and mine is in front of the TV on the couch eating junk food.

In some respects I did better than I would have expected. After three months of a very strict routine there are some things for which I have lost the taste. Among them is milk chocolate, which used to be a staple of my sitting on the couch in front of the TV routine. Instead, I switched to dark chocolate, a much healthier alternative. I can't even stand the taste of milk chocolate any more. Most meals during which I have meat, I go with chicken or turkey skipping red meat. One of my favorite hiatus meals was turkey sandwiches, but instead of the fat-filled mayo I grew up on I opted for mustard instead, a much better alternative. So from what I've told you so far, it doesn't sound so bad, right? Well there were also a few other items in the dietary rotation that weren't smart selections. Among my "why the hell did I eat that" items: ice cream (pounded down a quart on a few evenings), regular pizza (thick crust, extra cheese), fat-filled pasta (like lasagna), chips ('cause there's nothing better to do to a vegetable than deep fry it), and a couple reckless nights out ordering as I pleased from the menu. Needless to say I enjoyed my little break.

STUPID MISTAKES MADE ON HIATUS

I figured it would be easier to wrap up all the stupidity in one section, so here they are, in no particular order:

- Not controlling the length of the hiatus: confession here— this hiatus lasted three months, three glorious months. While I would say a hiatus is a good idea to keep you reaching for a long-term weight loss goal, letting that hiatus last three months isn't a good idea. How did it happen? Simple: I let it. I allowed one week to become a month to become a quarter of a year. Lack of control; go figure.

- Completely stopping exercise: this didn't happen in the first week or two, but by the end of the first month I was completely done exercising. Yep, done. Really bad idea. It will take weeks to get back on track now. I can imagine the pain I am going be in those first couple weeks. If you wander off the diet make sure you keep the exercise program going. I know I will in the future.

- Ignoring the numbers: for ninety days I didn't get on my scale, not once. Didn't write down what I was eating either; what's the point when you're ignoring your health? Besides, I was too busy stuffing my face to worry about writing down what I stuffed it with.

- Thinking I could magically eat whatever I want: one of my motivations for doing this was to address issues I had arising from food I ate. Basically my stomach couldn't handle my preferred menu selections. So what did I do on hiatus? I went right back to eating whatever I wanted; without regard to the effects it would have on my stomach. Those problems that got me here in the first place came right back.

What have I learned from these stupid mistakes? First, I learned I am a health idiot. No matter how much better I feel when eating right & exercising I will gladly trade that for garbage food. So in order to battle my own stupidity I need to keep myself on a strict plan. As long as I have a strong plan & work it I am fine; as soon as I let myself think I can be trusted when left to my own devices, I am a train wreck. Second, I learned that while hiatuses are necessary to a long-term process, they have to be controlled & limited. It was supposed to be a break, not a return to the fat old days. Third, I learned that even a health idiot like myself can make long-standing changes if I give it enough time. If Act Two creates some more minor changes, I will be well on my way to a healthy lifestyle by the beginning of our final act. Oh yeah, our little program here is going to be a three-act play. My plan is to stick to it for the next ten weeks (until Christmas, another great milestone, just like we had in Act

One with the trip to California) and then take a month-long hiatus before the last act, which will run until my twentieth high school reunion that June, again another big milestone. Notice the theme? Moving toward a visible goal with a clearly identifiable & personally meaningful ending point is a great way to keep you on track.

LESSONS LEARNED FROM ACT ONE

So what did I learn from Act One?

- Extreme calorie reduction diets, followed religiously & with the assistance of exercise actually work—probably shouldn't be a big surprise here, but we all see the endless commercials with spokespeople, both famous & not, spewing the values of the product they are paid to endorse. Well, if those programs are designed around eating at regular intervals, comprised of food with the right ingredients, heavily restrictive on calories, following the program religiously & introducing exercise into the mix, then yes they do work. You have to follow it religiously; if you can't, then save yourself the heartache & continue doing what you are doing until you are ready to make that kind of commitment.

- If you do go on a program I would highly recommend one where you don't have to consider too many options (I stuck with some shakes & bars & ate the same meal nightly, not a lot of thinking required in that equation). This way you can give your mind a chance to change the way it thinks about food. For Act Two, I won't be following the same program since I am looking to move to more of a real food, lifetime program so we will see what I can do on my own.

- Water is key: I was seriously surprised by how important water is, not only to weight loss but to general health. On my hiatus, one of the stupid things I did was not drink enough water. To take the weight off & keep your body moving & healthy you must drink enough water. How much is enough? That's a question that seems to produce different answers. I follow the half an ounce for every pound I weigh rule.

- Milestones keep you moving and tracking is essential: nothing keeps you on a diet like seeing the scale down a handful of pounds in a matter of days. Had I said, "Okay, I am going to drop one hundred pounds" & didn't break it down into manageable parts I would still be over three hundred pounds today. Tracking is very important and seeing progress is a great motivator. Also it allows you to fix any mistakes you may have made along the way by clearly identifying the results of your choices. So I say if you want to drop fifty pounds in six months, break it down per month & then per week. Keep yourself on track for the weekly goal by weighing yourself every couple days, that way you have plenty of time to right the ship if it goes off course.

CHAPTER FOUR

ACT TWO

GAME PLAN FOR ACT TWO

Act Two will be modeled after Act One, using bars and shakes and one regular meal, but the bars will be those readily available at stores and from various companies, and the regular meal will vary. Why modify something that's already worked?

- Availability: everything on the new plan will be readily available at most stores and not have to be ordered ahead of time.

- Higher daily calories: my goal for Act Two is to keep my daily caloric intake between 1200 and 1500.

- Lower expectations: over the next ten weeks I plan on getting down to 228. Right at the end of hiatus, I am probably around 250, so I am only looking to drop 22 pounds in the next ten weeks: 2.2 pounds a week.

- Didn't I mention I was hard–headed: this falls into the "having it my way" school of thought. Yes, I could continue the Act One program, but I want to see what I can come up with on my own. Basically I am looking for ownership of the program to give me a bit more motivation since I know going in I won't be seeing the huge pound drops I did in Act One.

ACT TWO: THE PROGRAM

The program for Act Two isn't dramatically different than Act One, more like a modified version. As mentioned I will be keeping the calorie intake to 1200 to 1500 a day, double what it was in Act One. Hopefully this is enough to allow me to expand my exercising, yet limiting enough to keep the weight coming off. The "real" meal of the day will vary but often will be the same as in Act One, but it won't always be dinner. I will be using a host of bars, all regularly available at superstores, drugstores, & grocery stores. What I am looking for in a bar: low calories (all bars will be less than two hundred calories), taste, high fiber, high protein, and low carbohydrates.

ACT 2

Day 1

Weight: 249.8

Weight gained from hiatus: 8.8 pounds

That's not so bad: gained less than nine pounds in ninety days. The basic healthy eating habits I did pick up must have countered enough of my own well-ingrained self-destructive eating habits to keep the gain to a minimum. Today was an easy day; my wife even mentioned I seemed fine on the diet. I reminded her that day one is easy; it's day three when it becomes a pain in the butt. I plan on popping on the scale on day three & better see a couple pounds gone for the sake of my own sanity. The bars today were pretty good; a couple actually tasted good. I felt a bit fuller today than I remember feeling in Act One. Of course, that could just be the residual effect of stuffing myself to the gills last night (a wonderful pre-diet ritual). The bars I am eating are high in fiber & I can feel it. Make sure, as I said before and especially if you are eating high-fiber bars, to drink lots & lots of water. Had the standby dinner: grilled chicken with romaine lettuce & some light dressing. Let the pound shedding begin!

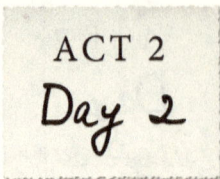

ACT 2

Day 2

Another relatively uneventful dietary day. There were a lot of them in Act One, so I guess we should plan on more of the same. I feel a bit more in "control" picking bars from among all offerings. As I said before, bar selection, as long as they fall into the low calorie, high fiber, high protein, low carbohydrate, is really just about taste & I have been pretty lucky picking good-tasting ones so far. The efforts large food companies have put into getting themselves a piece of the meal replacement bar market are really paying off for those of us whose diet is made up of mainly these; we can taste the fruits of their labor. We are lucky to be shedding our pounds in this day & age, because it is no longer acceptable to just have a nutritious & well-balanced meal replacement bar; if you want it to sell it had better taste good too. Dinner was the old fallback: grilled chicken & romaine lettuce with the extra special bonus of a half dozen pickle slices, 'cause I do like to live on the edge. These first two days dinner has tasted horrible. I got used to the palatable satisfaction pizza, pasta, & other carbohydrate-rich meals provide. Hopefully I get used to the dinner routine again; I don't remember the taste bothering me this much as Act One was coming to a conclusion; in fact, if I remember correctly, I was starting to like it. After two days I can already feel the increase in energy. My body is starting to clean out the junk & I can actually feel it, which is awesome; its reason alone to stick to this program, or at least that's what I keep telling myself. I haven't started exercising; I am planning on waiting until after week two to kick that into gear, which hopefully will deal successfully with any upcoming plateaus.

ACT 2
Day 3

Today I went on a hunt for more bar options. My hunting grounds were big bulk retailers & drugstores. Both had suitable bars, but the drugstore was more expensive; I guess you are paying for convenience. So I proved my point that the mixed bag of bars program would be easy to follow because of easy accessibility. Now for a caveat: there are a lot of bar options out there, & some aren't meal-replacement bars. Make sure the bars you buy to replace meals are actually meal-replacement bars. As far as the calories: most are under two hundred calories, protein heavy, & carbohydrate light. I did read some articles & blogs that knocked different bars for having ingredient issues, but let's be realistic: if you're like me & you ate yourself fat, whatever are in the bars isn't anywhere near as bad as what you consumed to pack on the pounds in the first place. So at the end of the day, no matter what Dr Zero Body Fat has to say about certain bars, we are actually eating healthier despite the criticized bar ingredients. That's one of the problems with dieting today: "health experts" have a lifetime of healthy eating & exercise behind them, married with genetic bless-ings, so they simply can't relate to those of us looking to drop some pounds without killing ourselves doing so. We aren't the people look-ing for perfectly sculpted abs; most of us would just be happy to be able to see our feet. So again bar selection, as long it meets the calorie, protein, & low carbohydrate parameters, is all about taste. Okay, off the soapbox; three days down.

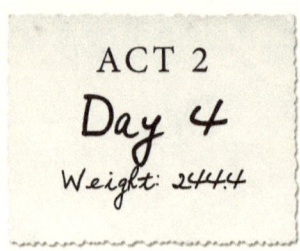

ACT 2

Day 4

Weight: 2444

Wow, that is a much bigger drop than I expected in three days. The wonders of fiber? The power of water? Most likely it is a combination of those factors & the reduction in daily calories. I am going to assume I was consuming three to four thousand calories a day on hiatus, & now I have cut that in at least half. Not rocket science: reduced calories equal reduced weight. I have managed to keep my sleep in the seven-hour-a-night range over the past three days; I hope I can keep that up. I know how important sleep is to weight loss & general health, but I have typically paid it as much mind as I have my diet—sure, it's the right thing to do, but the opposite is so much more fun.

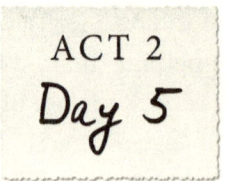

ACT 2

Day 5

Today was just another typical diet day. I feel obligated to provide a fiber-related warning: drink plenty of water. Based on my experience, the first four days you will be dehydrating quickly & often. I am not back to the .5 ounces for every pound rate yet but I am pretty close. Dehydration is pretty easy to see: basically, the darker your urine the more dehydrated you are. Today I did mix it up a bit and had a turkey sandwich for dinner. The bread helped settle my unhappy stomach. That is going to be key for Act Two: making adjustments based on what my body is telling me. I also added unsalted peanuts back into my dietary options. Hey, I am already at double what I was planning on losing this week, so I am playing with house money.

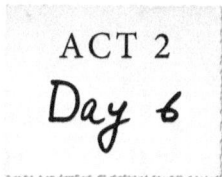

ACT 2
Day 6

More stomach troubles today; I am wondering when I will adapt to the high fiber. I will tell you I had stomach issues before I started dieting, so you may not have the same problems with the fiber-heavy diet, but at the very least you were warned. Had another turkey sandwich today, this time for lunch, & it seemed to help my stomach a bit.

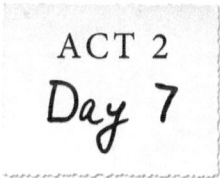

ACT 2
Day 7

Lazy day today. Well, it is a Sunday during football season so, come on, you can't expect too much activity. At some point I have to get back to exercising; I can feel the effects of my inactivity. The diet went pretty well today, with the exception of eating one too many bars & a few mouthfuls too many peanuts, but hey, I already passed the weekly goal, so why not live a little.

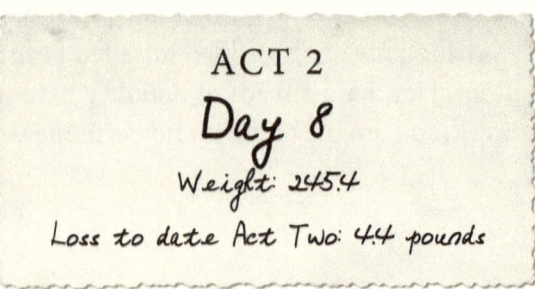

ACT 2

Day 8

Weight: 2454

Loss to date Act Two: 4.4 pounds

So looks like those extra mouthfuls of peanuts may have added up. Still, my goal is 21 pounds in 10 weeks, which is only 2.1 pounds a week, so I more than doubled that. As time goes on with this program, figuring out ways to adjust is key. Sure, I would love to order a pizza, but if I can accomplish the same thing with a four-hundred-calorie sandwich (which is the need to comfort-eat), it's a win, mainly because it will keep me on the program since I have a way of dealing with days that just demand something that tastes good as a reward, or, in this case, a comfort.

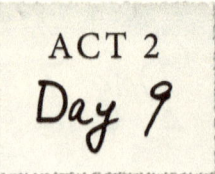

ACT 2

Day 9

Well I must admit without the structure of the Act One program, sticking to a diet is a lot rougher than I thought. When I am in charge of my diet choices, I get a lot of opportunities to make less than the best choices, & I am damn good at making poor food choices. So far it hasn't been anything horrific, but it also hasn't been the disciplined selections that made the weight fall off in Act One. Right now I am focusing on trying to get my sleep in line; one benefit of working for yourself is being able to set your own hours. The downside of that is that 4 AM is as likely a work hour as 4 PM, so keeping my sleep in line is yet another project.

ACT 2
Day 10

What the hell? 247.4! Seriously! I gained two pounds in two days? Sure, I haven't been completely strict with the diet, but I haven't been dining on pizza & washing it down with milkshakes either. Looking back over the past forty-eight hours of pound packing, I can see a few patterns. One is I have liberally snacked on crackers & cheese, so from now on that's out. I also added cheese to my turkey sandwich; sorry cheese, you are getting the boot again. I have gone through an ocean of soda, but the water bottles are relatively untouched. So clearly I need to make a few changes over the next couple days to get the scale moving in the right direction. All right. so back on track—well, not really today because I have a business dinner & eating out is almost a lost cause. I mean they have two-thousand-calorie salads on some menus. I tried to keep the damage to a minimum; that's about the best you can hope for when dining out. Maybe I will start walking again. I have been battling the first head cold of the winter for a couple weeks, but I might have to suck it up & beat my feet if I want to see progress.

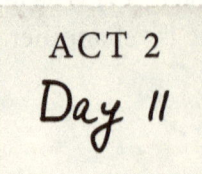

ACT 2

Day 11

It is amazing the effect eating has on your weight. Now I am not talking about the obvious situation of comparing a low-calorie diet to stuffing your face with pizza, chips, cookies, & ice cream (or, as I like to call it, my plans in heaven). I mean the little differences between a disciplined & structured diet (like Act One) & a slightly more flexible one. It's not like I spent the past couple days living at a buffet; I really only varied from the basics of Act One with a couple turkey sandwiches, some peanuts, & one dinner out. Wouldn't think that would start a scale surge. However I can't argue with the weight gain over the past couple days; the facts don't lie. I am still hoping to get back on track over the next ten days or so, but I am not sure if it will work.

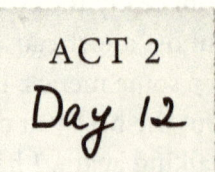

ACT 2

Day 12

Today was another dietary struggle. Sure, work related stress was a bit high, but there were stressful days during Act One too. Maybe the struggle has to do with not having enough of a well-defined event toward which I am racing. Maybe it's the fact that I am not going after a fifty-pound plus drop, but rather a mere twenty pounds. Maybe I am just lazy; always a possibility. I am beginning to discover why highly structured diet programs have such a high success rate & why so many people struggle on their own. Taking thought out of the equation & just eating as ordered does make life a lot easier.

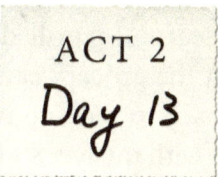

ACT 2

Day 13

Really bad diet day today. My wife made some banana bread & I couldn't get enough. The reason I am failing in Act Two might be too many carbohydrates. I am not looking forward to weight day tomorrow; I know I won't be happy with what I see on the scale. Again, not that I have been horrible this week: sure I went out to dinner once, oh & got pizza with my wife, & the banana bread, & a couple boxes of crackers with cheese, &, oh hell, I guess it was a bad week. While none of those things alone in a week are horrible, when you add it all up over seven days it can be a nuclear assault of your dietary goals. I have to figure a way to make changes that will get the weight loss ball rolling again.

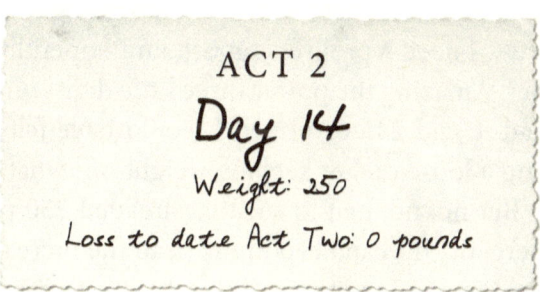

ACT 2

Day 14

Weight: 250

Loss to date Act Two: 0 pounds

I knew the scale wasn't going to be good, but I didn't expect to gain back all the weight I had managed to lose in Act Two. Two weeks in & nothing to show for it: that's encouraging. I spent today researching where I am going wrong & I really think it has to do with carbohydrates. So I went & got some melba thin seedless rye bread, which has half the calories & carbohydrates as the sourdough I had been eating. I won't be having pizza, crackers, cheese, or banana bread this week. I picked up some more unsalted peanuts to snack on, a host of bars to choose from, & grilled chicken. Let's see if forty bucks of the right stuff at the grocery can get me back on track. I am dedicated to getting back to walking next week, even spent the ten bucks on stuff to deal with my feet so I can manage a few miles without breaking into tears—as a man I prefer to cry once I get safely in my home out of sight of the neighbors. Well, any journey begins with the first step so I am taking first, or more accurately retaking my first step now.

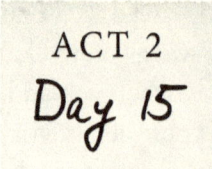

ACT 2

Day 15

The calorie count today was most likely in the 1200-range; that ought to do the trick, at least in theory. I am going to jump on the scale tomorrow. I need a progress report, and hopefully I will see a better number. Amazing the power three little digits on a scale have over you. Had it said 245 or under, I would have felt like the big winner: eating a loose diet & keeping weight off; what more could you ask for? But no, no, had to see that dreaded 250 pounds. I do feel more energetic. If I can keep in my head the increase in energy I feel when on the diet I may actually be able to stay on it—again, at least in theory.

ACT 2
Day 16

Amazing: 245! Couldn't ask for more: five pounds in two days; doesn't even seem possible. If anything, I have learned in this little experiment that the scale is a strange mistress. Over the past two days the winning weight loss combination has been: under-150-calorie bars, coffee, water, turkey & mustard sandwiches on thin rye, and peanuts. Not a bad diet but I don't know how long I can keep to that restrictive menu. I did pick up some sub hundred-calorie snack bars that at least offer a variety as far as taste is concerned. I even took a couple to the movies today; let me warn you some of them open loudly—I mean really loudly—and they don't always travel well, so be prepared to either lick the bulk of them out of the wrapper or go without. Good thing for me I am not too proud to lick a wrapper.

ACT 2
Day 17

It seems my stomach is adjusting to the high fiber content, which should keep my marriage intact. Seriously you have to be careful with the fiber, trust me. I am still not drinking enough water, which isn't good when you are consuming a lot of fiber. Other than that I would say this week has been a success. Hopefully I can get down to around 242 or 243 by this coming Monday's weigh-in, undoing all my self-induced damage from the prior off week. The variety of bars and the ability to snack on peanuts is helping; at least there is a little variety and I am getting enough calories to prevent me from passing out, so far.

ACT 2
Day 18

I picked up more bars and some things to treat my feet; the thing that sucks about being sedentary for so long is it takes a real toll on your body when you do finally decide to get off your lazy butt. I also had to pick up candy for Halloween. What kind of holiday encourages kids to gorge on candy and then make us adults suffer with the remains of what we couldn't distribute? We had thought about passing out something healthy, but who wants to clean egg off the front of the house? Luckily I got out of a party invitation since we couldn't leave the dog alone with kids coming to the door. Not that I don't like parties, but I have a little over eight weeks to drop another seventeen pounds, so I don't really have the wiggle room to pig out on party food. Sure I could exercise self-control, but let's be honest I have yet to show I know anything about self-control. It took about three weeks for me to adjust to the program in Act One and I am figuring it will take about the same length of time in Act Two. Three weeks is a generic time frame that you will often hear is the length of time it will take a person to adjust to something.

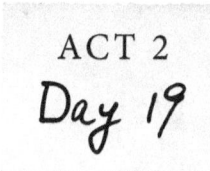

ACT 2

Day 19

Oh, the joy of Halloween: passing out candy to help advance childhood obesity and then getting left with half a bowl of undistributed junk. What a joy. Luckily one of my neighbors has kids, so I can pass the remains off. Well, most of them, but how bad can a "fun size" bar be? It's fun sized, and fun is good, right? Are you seeing how I managed to get myself a hundred pounds overweight? The rest of the day went as planned. I even increased my water consumption a good amount; still not drinking enough but its progress. So Halloween is over, which symbolizes the kick off of the holiday season. This will be my first holiday season trying to live healthy, and I already know it is going to be a challenge.

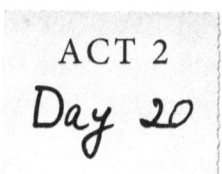

ACT 2

Day 20

Halloween followed by a Sunday of football: how exactly am I supposed to follow a diet? Well I did, as well as possible—at least today. I have been craving pizza; I have to figure out a way to get that into this week. I was thinking I could have some once I get to 240, setting that as the next milestone. Right now I am just hoping the scale is in the 242-range tomorrow.

ACT 2
Day 21
Weight: 244.4

Loss to date Act Two: 5.6 pounds

I will take the five-plus pound loss. I made up for my bad week and am within range of 240, or as we will now call it "pizza weight." Hopefully I can get down to 240 soon because how much longer can I put off the need for pizza. Seriously, it is a *need*. Didn't start exercising today like I was supposed to; I am going to go with the "got busy at work" excuse. Yeah, that's a good one: I got too busy with work to find thirty minutes to walk; that makes perfect sense. Hopefully I can either manage to exercise or find myself a better excuse tomorrow. Another good diet day; I think I am settling in, although I still have massive cravings, cravings I didn't have before I ended Act One. This will be tougher since I am not going to see the massive weekly loses as I did in Act One so I had better prepare myself—not that I have any idea how to do that, other than constantly repeating, *It's progress, it's progress,* in my head over and over and hitting my milestones.

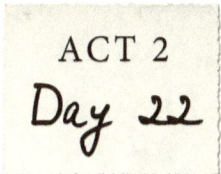

ACT 2

Day 22

So I seem to be struggling to motivate myself to work out. It is amazing how once you get off track it is so hard to get back on it. I know this will catch up to me on the scale. Otherwise diet went pretty well; so far I have been able to control my cravings. I will say they seem stronger in Act Two now that I have "control" over my menu selections. So far I have resisted, but the week is young.

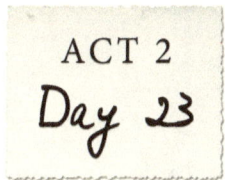

ACT 2

Day 23

All right, so my string of days without working out continues. I am shocked at how hard it is to get back to it. Today I had a different excuse: we went to dinner to celebrate a career victory for my wife. Yeah, who needs exercise when you can have food? But at least I had a better excuse, right? Anyway, to wrap up the day of no exercise and a poor diet selection for dinner; maybe I need to throw myself on the scale tomorrow?

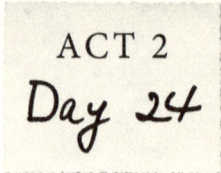

ACT 2
Day 24

The facts don't lie: I hit 245.5 today. Twenty-three days down and I have managed to lose 4.5 pounds. That isn't a very good trend. So did I start exercising today? Of course not; that would make way too much sense. I did stick to a low-calorie diet, but somehow I don't think that is enough—or at least is hasn't been. Maybe I am eating more calories than I think. I better start keeping better track. Hopefully I can make a small dent in the weight before Monday's scale day so this week isn't a complete loss.

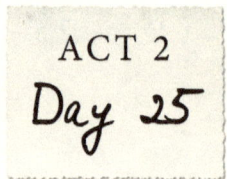

ACT 2
Day 25

Shocker here for you: another day without exercise. I know, I know you are amazed. My excuse for the day…well, I don't have one. At this point, I figure I might as well put off until Monday what I should have started last week. Monday I plan to force myself out there for a half-hour walk, no matter what. The diet went okay today, but I still am not drinking enough water and eating too many calories. It's the peanuts that are killing me; I mean I would know if I were to track it, but I haven't gotten myself to that point yet.

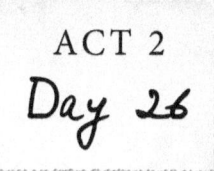

ACT 2
Day 26

I needed the protein. That doesn't sound like a bad excuse, right? Well, how about if I give you the full picture: we ordered light sauce, light cheese, thin crust pizza for movie night tonight, and since I needed the protein I ordered a side of spicy chicken wings. Chicken is good for you, right? Yeah, maybe wing isn't the best form of chicken, but some protein is better than none. Sure, I could have eaten the precooked grilled chicken I had in the fridge, but who doesn't love wings? Sadly, the spicy wings kicked my butt and I had to eat a sleeve of crackers to calm my stomach down; that sounds like a pretty bad excuse, too. Is it Monday yet?

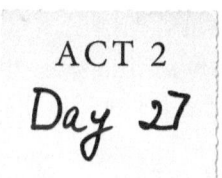

ACT 2
Day 27

Tomorrow is scale day; oh, this should be so much fun. I am thinking the scale will be around 248 tomorrow morning, based on how poorly I ate this week. Seeing as how I am either going to have to give up on losing weight or really bunker down, we decided to go out with a bang and order pizza a second night in a row—this time no chicken wings, though. Come tomorrow I will be tracking every calorie I take in, pouring water down my throat, and working out, no matter what.

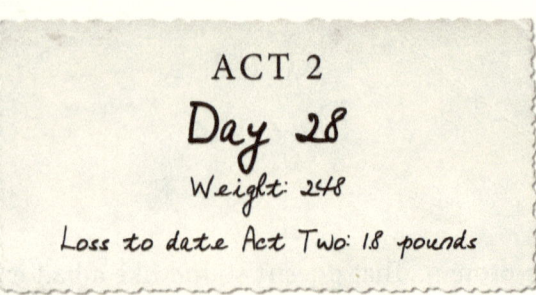

ACT 2
Day 28
Weight: 248
Loss to date Act Two: 18 pounds

Well four weeks and I managed to drop almost a whole two pounds. Seriously, time to buckle down, *today*. Actually, more like four weeks ago, but since my time machine isn't perfected yet, I'd better start today. I am diligently writing down everything I eat; today I had a total of 950 calories, which consisted of five bars and a turkey sandwich on rye. If I can keep this up I should be able to lose weight. It was likely the snacking that killed me—that and the lack of exercise. So I also got back into the walking today, and let me tell you it wasn't the least painful experience. If I was a smarter man I would have never stopped walking, but then this story wouldn't be as interesting. Going forward, the plan is 1000 calories a day and walking every day for thirty minutes; assuming I am not completely cursed I should be down under 245 by the end of this week.

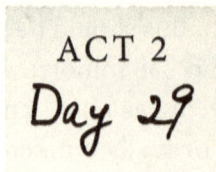

ACT 2
Day 29

Day two of walking, and my legs are killing me. Hopefully by the end of the week I should be back to being able to make it through the walk without huffing or puffing. Another successful day on the diet: again stuck to under 1000 calories, and the second time around adjusting to such a low amount of calories is just as hard as the first time. Even had a couple of the light-headed spells; aren't they fun. Going to sneak onto the scale tomorrow, and at this point I am just hoping it's moving in the right direction.

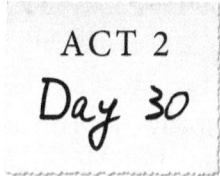

ACT 2

Day 30

243.6! Hot damn, I am moving in the right direction. I really can't complain about dropping 4.4 pounds in two days. So I guess keeping the calories under 1000 and actually getting off my lazy butt works. Of course today I felt like I got run over by a train; maybe I am pushing it a bit too much. Given the loss I have so far I took today off from exercising; in fact I did very little today that required any movement.

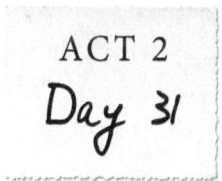

ACT 2

Day 31

Wow, did I feel better today. I had a ton of energy all day, even took a nice long walk in the cold rain. I am adjusting again to the reduced calories; hopefully I don't see too many more days where I hit the wall.

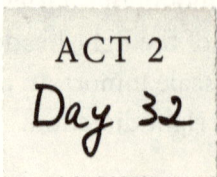

ACT 2

Day 32

Snuck onto the scale today: still 243.6. Guess that walk yesterday was for nothing. Hopefully this is just one of those phases where the scale doesn't change for a day or two and then I see a couple pounds fall off. I didn't get a chance to walk today—actually, let me correct myself: I opted not to walk today, figuring I can do it tomorrow when the weather is supposed to be nicer. It was another successful diet day, so hopefully that will pay off in a couple days when I weigh in for the week.

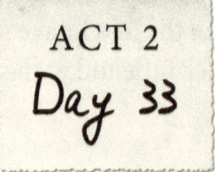

ACT 2

Day 33

All right, I got the walk today, which should make up for yesterday. I drove the path I walk so I could figure the distance, and it is a whole two miles. I was thinking it was a lot more. So Monday I am going to up it to three and a half miles. That would put me at half a 10K, assuming it doesn't kill me. Diet went well today, but it was harder to follow than most days, and a lot harder than I wish it were. Oh well, one day left till I get on the scale.

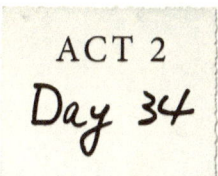

ACT 2

Day 34

Sunday may be the toughest day of the week for me. Maybe it is because I tend to spend Sundays in front of the television watching football, which is packed full with food commercials. Maybe I ought to go get myself a hobby, or throw the remote through the TV. If I am going to make it through until Christmas and actually manage to shed those last pounds I better come up with something. No walk today—you know, because I was busy watching football and the food commercials.

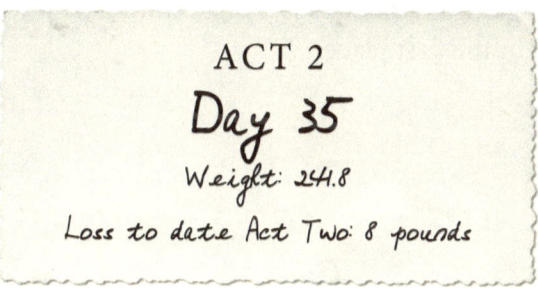

ACT 2

Day 35

Weight: 244.8

Loss to date Act Two: 8 pounds

Now that's a lot better! Over six pounds in a week; what more could I ask for? I am almost back to the lowest weight I have seen, and am fewer than five pounds away from once again entering unchartered territory. I managed to walk three and a half miles today, and did it in forty-two minutes. I have to get the distance and per-mile time up to be able to actually complete a 10K before the finish line is packed away, but at least I am out there again. My plan going forward is cardio one day and weights the next. I can see myself getting back to the 237-range by next week if I keep to the workout schedule and don't venture off the diet.

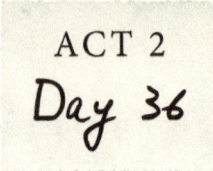

ACT 2

Day 36

Did weights today, and boy do I feel it. There is nothing like the feeling of going back to weight training after taking a couple months off—and by that I mean the feeling of pure pain. Everything that can hurt does. Guess this is the price I pay for that hiatus. Assuming I remember this pain come the next hiatus maybe I won't stop working out just because I allow myself some diet liberty—which isn't a guarantee, otherwise I probably wouldn't have stopped working out during the first hiatus since I had similar pain when I started working out in the first place.

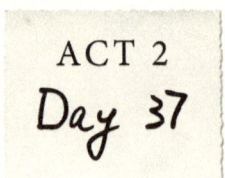

ACT 2

Day 37

What the hell: 241! I actually gained weight eating less than a thousand calories a day and doing weights and cardio? How is that even possible? I was hoping it was just a scale error, so I took the batteries out and retried: nope, still 241. My wife kindly tried the "maybe it's muscle added from the weight lifting" line but come on, one day of weight training isn't going to put a pound of muscle on, especially since the weight I am lifting is unimpressive at best. Did another 5K today; I figure if I can do a 5K every other day for the next couple weeks I should be able to start increasing the distance until I get to the seven-mile mark in preparation for the official 10K I plan on doing.

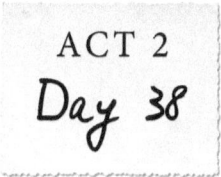

ACT 2

Day 38

Ouch. That is about all I have to say today: ouch. Everything hurts worse than the days before. I did no working out at all today, didn't even put my fat butt on the scale because I don't think I can deal with bad news and this much pain in one day. Seriously, even my fingers hurt; how is that even possible? One tough thing about dieting is the celebratory aspect of food. Both my wife and I had big work successes this week, but we had to forgo the typical dinner out in celebration because of this damn diet. So we skipped it and instead decided to wait until the scale went under 240 for me.

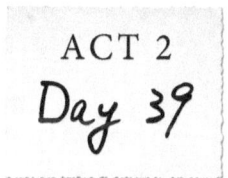

ACT 2

Day 39

Finally a number under 240: weight today was 239! It is about time; I was getting nervous, debating between returning to the program I used in Act One and seeking liposuction (which I regularly consider anyway). We opted to do that celebratory dinner as pizza and a movie at home and went with the thin crust, light sauce, and light cheese pizza hoping it doesn't kill my success this week. I really want to see that scale at or under 237 come Monday. Got my 5K in; time is still an issue, seeing as it took me forty-five minutes, but I guess I shouldn't be too hard on myself since I just started. Besides, I finally broke back below 240! All in all a great day.

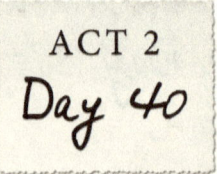

ACT 2

Day 40

Got back to weights today; didn't even think about putting my pizza-stuffed face on the scale. The pain isn't so bad, especially if I get on the scale tomorrow and still see a sub-240 number. My reasoning for weighing myself tomorrow is simple: if the number is bad I can increase my cardio and hopefully get it close to the 237 I wanted for this week. Once I break the 237-barrier I will again be entering unchartered territory and I can't wait! It amazes me to think I haven't seen this type of weight in like two decades, and I'm not even forty. Thankfully I finally made my health a priority; hopefully I can keep at it.

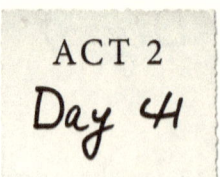

ACT 2

Day 41

All right, what the hell: the scale said 241 today! I gained two pounds in two days and I did both a 5K and weight training during those two days. There is no way that should even be possible, so I went searching for reasons online. In reading a couple dozen articles I found a theory that weight training can make the scale go up; muscles expand and hold more water and that it is normal to see the scale change a couple pounds here and there. On one site the "expert" was going on about how scales aren't important, and then he discloses he has never been one to struggle with body fat or weight. Here is the thing: unless you have been a fat person, don't tell us what a scale means! A scale is one indicator of whether we are doing the right things or not. We need every indicator moving in the right direction, because to us we aren't simply reducing calories; we are starving ourselves, depriving ourselves of one of our favorite pleasures: food. On the upside, I was able to add something to the menu: fried egg sandwiches, sort of. I fry two eggs using a no-calorie cooking spray, and put them over one English muffin. It totals about 300 calories, so it is well within the low-calorie guidelines I am trying to follow. I had one a day for the last two days and I must say it does give me a bit of an energy boast, and it is nice to eat something different. Let's hope the scale is back under 240 tomorrow, otherwise I might have to take drastic measures—as soon as I figure out what would be more drastic than what I have been doing.

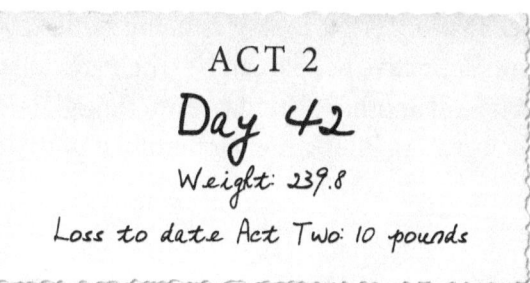

ACT 2

Day 42

Weight: 239.8

Loss to date Act Two: 10 pounds

That just may be the toughest ten pounds anyone has ever lost. It makes me long for the weeks of five- and six-pound losses; of course there was a lot more to lose back then. Today was cardio; my plan this week is two days of cardio, one day of weights, followed by two days of cardio. Hopefully that will get the weight down to 236 by the end of this week. They say losing two pounds a week is healthy, but come on, I can still see plenty that needs to go. Besides, I think I have earned a five-pound drop.

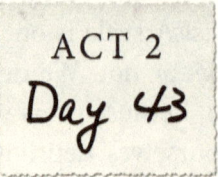

ACT 2

Day 43

Well this Thursday is Thanksgiving, the ultimate "make a pig out of yourself" holiday. The food options are endless, in massive quantities, and everywhere you go you are reminded of the feast coming up. This Thanksgiving we are going nontraditional: a barbeque chicken pizza, with thin crust, light sauce, light cheese, and extra chicken. Yeah, I know, not what most people want to see on their Thanksgiving Day table. We are obviously skipping all those fattening but oh-so-good desserts. Hopefully I don't fall off track. I scheduled a couple meetings for next week, and while these are the type of meetings you would usually have over lunch I got both parties to agree to coffee instead. All it took was being honest; you would be surprised how supportive people can be when you tell them you are on a strict diet. I did another 5K today, even though it was cold, a bit rainy, and my feet were killing me. Hopefully it pays off.

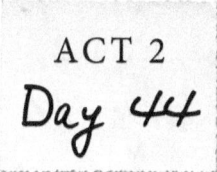

ACT 2

Day 44

I got an off day from cardio & spent it lifting weights instead—don't I know how to party. I am starting to see some effect from the weight lifting, both in my strength and a bit in my body shape. Of course I don't look like I am ready for a remake of the movie *300*, but I look a lot better than when I started. At this point I can't wait until tomorrow to have something different for dinner; sure there won't be any pie but at least it will be something different.

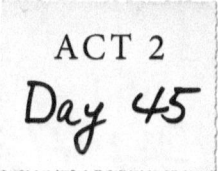

ACT 2

Day 45

Thanksgiving: the greatest holiday on an overeater's calendar. It's that rare day when it is generally acceptable to participate in eating like a pig. Sadly, I couldn't play my usual snout-wearing role this year. Instead, we had barbeque chicken pizza with thin crust, very light sauce and cheese, and extra chicken and it was awesome. It is amazing the foods that taste so good when you are denying yourself everything. I did another 5K today. A neighbor asked me if I was walking off my holiday feast; if she only knew how long it's been since I feasted. I actually managed to jog a bit today; wow, has it been a long time since I have done that. I felt it in my knee and ankle, so I didn't over-do it since I have to hit the road again tomorrow but it is a start.

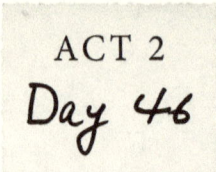

ACT 2

Day 46

Another day of cardio; the scale showed no ill effects from my un-traditional Thanksgiving Day feast; it actually went down about 1.5 pounds, which means I should be able to hit the two-pound mark by Monday's weigh-in. I even treated myself to leftover pizza from yesterday; hey, I figure I earned it. Did a little more jogging today; I don't know how long it will take before I can jog the entire 5K; at this rate, maybe this time three years from now but the scale is moving in the right direction and at least I am doing cardio.

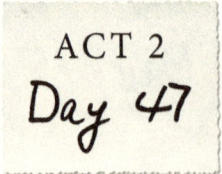

ACT 2

Day 47

Another day of hitting the weights. I added a couple things based on that pile of magazines on fitness that have been gathering on my bathroom floor. I worked my abs extra hard, not in anticipation of having a six-pack, but rather to look a little less Santa-like. Went and bought some clothes today, since things seem to not be fitting. Before I began Act One (less than six months ago), I bought a pair of jeans that were a 44-inch waist; today I bought a pair that is a 36-inch waist! An added bonus: right before I began this journey I was a size 3-X shirt; today I am a large. My wife kept saying I look so much better but I didn't believe it until I picked up those jeans. I must say buying such a smaller size makes clothes shopping enjoyable. These results make this long torturous journey bearable! Hopefully the scale is in the 237-range tomorrow; otherwise I am going to have to grab a day of cardio when I had planned on taking tomorrow off completely.

ACT 2
Day 48

Great day today: scale said 237 so I took a day off from working out. As an added bonus for my ego I tried on the clothes I wore right before I started Act One; let me tell you, that was a wonderful feeling. I can't believe they actually fit at one point. It is hard to believe the difference between a size 44-inch waist pants and a size 36. My wife was happy I finally got it through my thick skull that I look a lot better. Putting on the old shirt and pants was something else. My plan is to keep on the same plan for the next twenty-six days, increasing the exercise along the way and then figure out a way to make Act Three's diet more regular food and fewer bars, because the high fiber and low everything else is killing me. I did some research on daily calorie burn and based on a calculator I found online I should be taking in 3200 to 3500 calories a day to maintain my weight. One of the simplest concepts of weight loss is that one pound equals 3500 calories, so if you want to lose a pound a week, eat 3500 calories less than you burn. Since I aim to drop two pounds a week I need to eat 7000 calories less than I use in a week, or 1000 calories less a day. I figure in Act Three I should be able to consume 2000 calories of regular food a day and still drop around two pounds a week, assuming I keep my exercise level high and incorporate more activity into my regularly sedentary work routine.

ACT 2

Day 49

Weight: 239.6

Loss to date Act Two: 10.2 pounds

There is no way possible I could have added two and a half pounds in twenty-four hours. I am going to assume today was just a screwy scale day and hop back on tomorrow morning. This type of diet makes me basically a raw nerve, so everything seems to be irritating me, including an uncooperative scale. Today I was drained; just seemed to have no gas in the tank. Of course as a cruel act of irony I have plenty of other gas from the high fiber diet. I took the walk up to four miles today; maybe that will jump-start the scale again. Act Three is all about figuring out a way to eat real food; well, real *healthy* foods. The last act becomes a permanent change to my diet, because there is no way I could stay on this for the rest of my life and if I don't figure out a way to eat regular food healthy than I will pack all that weight right back on.

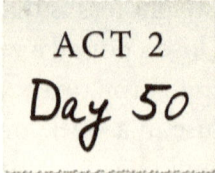

ACT 2

Day 50

Good day on the scale today: 236.4. Sadly, that prompted me to do absolutely no exercise today. Sure I had a busy day, plenty of meetings and activity, but come on, I easily could have found thirty minutes to get a walk in. It is almost like I reward myself for success on the scale by making sure there will be disappointment on it later. Figuring out the right protein bar formula has been a real challenge; I had to eat some crackers today just to settle my stomach enough so I could sleep. My plan tomorrow is to do both cardio and weights, since that clock is ticking on me.

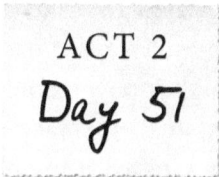

ACT 2

Day 51

All right, well at least today I was able to get in both the cardio and the weights. Did another four miles today, and I felt every inch of it. It might take me a while to get to the seven miles I need to hit to be 10K ready, but I will get there. It does amaze me how much knees, ankles, and feet can hurt. I did the cardio early and the weights at night. Now there are hundreds of articles on which to do first, how to do both the same day, how you shouldn't do both the same day, etc., but here is my thinking: since my primary goal is weight loss I figured the cardio is the most important, so I did that first, in case I didn't get to the weights. Tomorrow I will jump on the scale again, hoping that the number I see is no higher than 236.

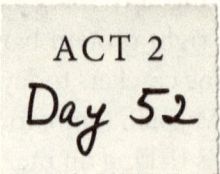

ACT 2

Day 52

So the scale gave me 237; I guess I will have to live with that. What are my choices, toss the scale? Then how would I torture myself? Got another four miles in today, again back to just walking it; trust me, that was painful enough today. Hopefully my cardio keeps improving to the point that I can increase my distance to 4.6 miles next week. So far I am sticking with my plan: get the distance over seven miles then start worrying about the time. I mean, it wasn't like I planned on giving the Kenyans a run for their money when I did a 10K. I really just want to be able to finish; that in itself would be a major accomplishment for me.

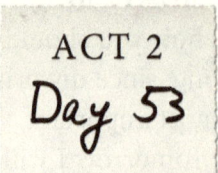

ACT 2

Day 53

Today was a pretty busy day, but I still managed to stick to the diet and get my weight training in, a major accomplishment considering how easily I could have let myself off the hook. Despite tweaking my elbow a bit, I managed to keep going and get a full workout in, even more impressive considering there are few better excuses than an injury. The diet seems like second nature: I again scheduled what were once lunch meetings over coffee. Once I have more information, do more research, and increase my self-control, I will be able to handle a lunch or dinner out, but until that happens I am the best advocate for my local coffee shop. One of those meetings yielded a pleasant surprise when we discussed the diet during that initial ice-breaking time. The person was almost floored when I shared that I spent most of my adult life over three hundred pounds. It is nice to see that sincere look of surprise in people's eyes. Who am I kidding—nice is an understatement. It's awesome!

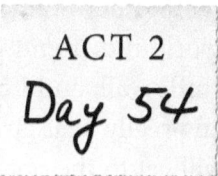

ACT 2

Day 54

The scale cooperated today: 236.8, so no complaints here. I am slowly adjusting to the idea that the scale will move in smaller and smaller increments as I get thinner and thinner, so I try to be positive from any small improvement. Took the day off from working out today, as the cold has really made it tough on my aches and pains. This has been an odd experience: after not giving a crap about what I looked like for most of my life, I now find myself suffering through body image issues that rival those of a fourteen-year-old girl. You would think I would be happy with the improvements to date, but no, I always wander back to noticing the flaws and the work I have left to do. Hopefully I will get over that soon enough; otherwise I might have to get some paint for my mirrors.

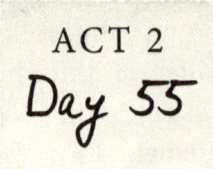

ACT 2

Day 55

Well this was a unique Sunday: I actually did cardio and weight training instead of spending yet another Sunday on the couch watching football. Amazingly the world didn't end, so I guess that theory of mine is shot. I did a four-mile walk and I can tell you all those extra pounds I carried for so long really beat up my joints. Hopefully, as I continue working out, I will get to the point where there will be less pain. I can't say that the pain has decreased as I have been working out, but then again the cold weather probably isn't helping. Another day of eating around 1200 calories; this better pay off tomorrow on the scale. I am hoping for somewhere in the 235-range.

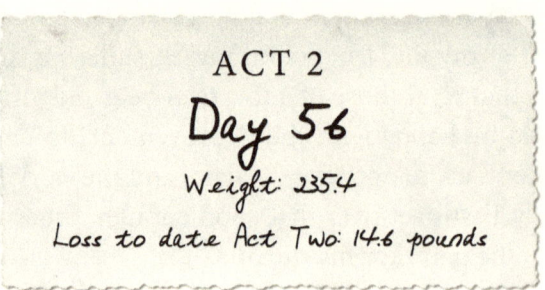

ACT 2

Day 56

Weight: 235.4

Loss to date Act Two: 14.6 pounds

Now that was a nice number to see on the scale this morning. It couldn't have come at a better time, since the last thing I wanted to do today was drag my aching body 4.6 miles in the cold, but seeing that number helped motivate me to do it. Eight weeks to lose 14.6 pounds is not really impressive, considering the weight loss I had in Act One. One of the things about losing weight is when you have so much less to lose, that extra weight is a lot more determined to stick with you. Based on my guesstimate I have maybe another twenty to twenty-five pounds I want to lose and we know that last twenty won't go away easily. We put up the Christmas tree today. This is a tough time of year to restrict your diet. My first thought after we got done was, *Time for cookies and eggnog.* Well obviously for me, no such luck. I instead had a protein bar and a glass of water—there is no way to paint that as an adequate substitution.

ACT 2
Day 57

It amazes me how easy it is to get so caught up in the things that occur in life that exercising no longer becomes a priority. Today was a typical example: I had to get a new laptop and setting it up sucked up the time I was originally going to spend working out. In fact I spent so much time setting up the new computer that I could only find time to order a pizza. There is always time to order a pizza, even on those days when you don't have time to exercise. Of course being so technologically stupid, it did take me quite a while to get everything up and running, but still I could have found time to eat right or exercise, rather than getting skipping my workout and ordering pizza. We were watching the finale of one of those popular weight-loss shows when something threw me. They focused solely on the scale, not the body fat percentage changes or overall fitness improvement. One guy, who lost, looked in much better shape than the guy who won. As I ranted about this (all the while chewing on pizza–oh the irony) my wife sat there snickering. Eventually I was able to figure out what she found so funny. It seems I have been doing the exact same thing. When she tells me how much better I look all I do is talk about the scale. This got me to thinking, *How can we more accurately measure our health?* You can get one of those fat pinchers that supposedly measures body fat, but how accurate can that be, and besides, who wants to pinch their fat first thing in the morning? There is a water-submersion test that measures body fat but that thing costs a couple hundred bucks a pop so how often are you going to do that? The best I have come up with as a working point is using measurements. If the scale stays the same but my arms are an inch bigger and my waist is an inch smaller, am I not in better health?

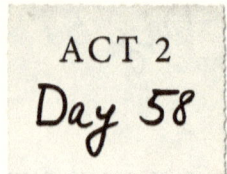

ACT 2

Day 58

Today I made up for my lazy day yesterday, finding time for weights and cardio despite the cold rain. Of course I had the additional motivation of the scale saying 237 this morning. No exercise, poor eating, and boom: the pounds come rolling back. Hopefully I can get back on track and get the scale moving back down in the next couple days. At the end of Act Two I am going to take measurements again and see how much I have improved from the very beginning. The scale is way too addicting and it creates such an emotional roller coaster; if I can add another measuring stick that is more stable it should help keep me off that roller coaster, in theory at least.

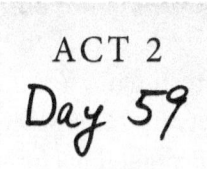

ACT 2

Day 59

So one good day, and then today hit. I did eat right but didn't find time to exercise at all. The four and a half mile goal is actually doing more harm than good. I could have easily found time to take a quick thirty-minute walk and two miles is better than no miles. So from now on, instead of focusing on the distance I am just going to focus on getting my lazy butt out there. It is amazing how easy it is to overcomplicate things to the point that you end up not doing the thing you overcomplicated in the first place, so tomorrow I am going to walk and work out, regardless of the time or distance. I am just going to do it. Also tomorrow is the wife's company holiday party, a fully-catered affair. It ought to be quit the test for me; let's hope I can at least manage a C-grade, might have to create a bell curve for this one.

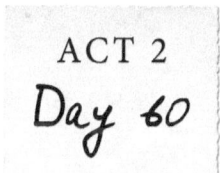

ACT 2

Day 60

Company Christmas parties are always interesting events, even more interesting when you add being on a strict diet to the mix. The food and alcohol were both in massive supply. I don't drink so that wasn't the source of temptation for me, but the endless amount of good-looking food—that's a different story. Overall I think I did really well. My plan was to stick to the healthier options and not stack the plate. They had the typical buffet eight-inch plates so I made sure I only used a quarter of it at any time to keep the quantity of whatever I was eating in check. I stuck to the fresh fruit and vegetables; wow have I missed fresh fruit. You forget how good strawberries taste until you go a few months without them. Act Three's diet will include fresh fruit and vegetables for sure. After a couple hours I had a turkey sandwich and finished the night off with three small cookies; hey, it *is* a holiday party after all. Prior to the party I found the time to work out, although at a much quicker pace than normal since I was in a bit of a time crunch. Oh and did I mention the scale today said 235? One nice thing about the party is nobody I met there believed I use to weigh over three hundred pounds; it came up repeatedly as I passed on the assortment of "pack the pounds on" offerings and through my wife's bragging of my success. I am going to have to load some fat pictures on my phone so people can see that yes, I was well over three hundred pounds earlier this year. Looking at the pictures we took at the party it is amazing how different I look. There is no obvious belly hanging over the belt in the pictures of my side profile, which is a first for me. I actually have to admit I look pretty good, even though I still have a lot more work to do.

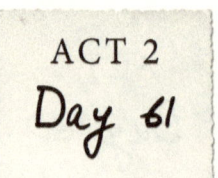

ACT 2

Day 61

It was freezing cold today, so no exercise; the pain I had just didn't make it a possibility. This type of bone-chilling cold isn't typical in the Southeast so I hope it passes quickly. My diet today wasn't great, nothing horrible but I didn't really stick to strict to anything; basically it was a miserable day. The pictures from last night's party probably made it a little easier for me to loosen up the diet. It amazes me that I don't see that guy in the pictures; instead, I still see the fatso I was a mere seven months ago. I guess it will take a while before how I see myself and reality match up.

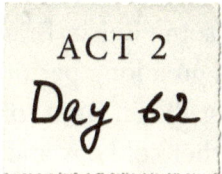

ACT 2

Day 62

Well it was cold and rainy again so no cardio but I did manage to get some weight training in. The cold made weight training a bit rough on the joints, but the point is I got it done, even though today is Sunday, and you know by now that Sundays and activity don't usually go together for me. No scale this morning: I didn't want to depress myself, and I figure I can wait until tomorrow and hope it is still in the 235-range, which considering the past couple days I will have to declare a victory. I kept to the diet today, most likely in a subconscious attempt to influence the scale tomorrow morning.

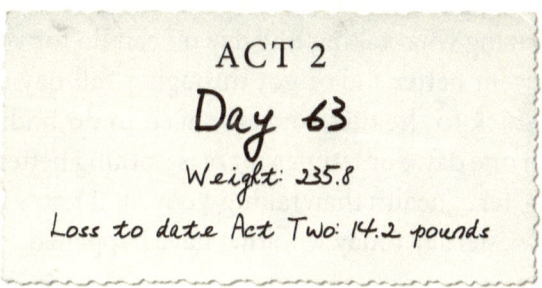

ACT 2

Day 63

Weight: 235.8

Loss to date Act Two: 14.2 pounds

Well wasn't that a waste of a week. I have come to the realization that I am going to wake up Christmas morning right around 235 and that is going to have to be okay. Really, what other options do

I have? That is the tough part about keeping on a diet when the weight isn't falling off half a dozen pounds at a time; it doesn't seem worth it to suffer so much considering the small rewards you can expect. If nothing else Act Two has taught me the importance of having a normal diet with regular foods as the weight continues to come off slowly in Act Three. So to compensate myself for a wasted week I treated myself to some Raisin Bran; it is amazing what you end up craving once you go a long period of time without regular food. I have been craving Raisin Bran for weeks. I skipped working out today; it was another cold day and I felt miserable, partially because of the weather and probably partially because of my scale failure. I figured why do today what I can put off until tomorrow?

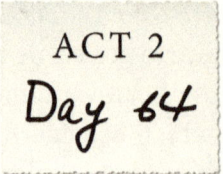

ACT 2

Day 64

Today went much better: got both cardio and weight training in and stuck to the diet. My plan is to walk again tomorrow then toss myself on the scale the following day and see if I am making progress. It is amazing what taking one day off can do for you. I felt one hundred percent better today, got through a full day of work and then some, stuck to the diet, and managed to do both cardio and weights all in one day. Sometimes there is nothing better you can do for your long-term health than taking a day off. I know if I hadn't let myself slack yesterday today wouldn't have happened.

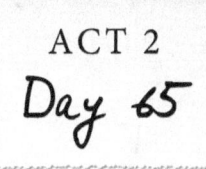

ACT 2

Day 65

Wow has the cold hit my part of the world. I did manage to get in four miles today, but it is getting harder and harder as the temperature goes down. This week is supposed to be a cold one so I have to find myself some inside cardio equipment ASAP.

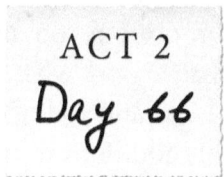

ACT 2

Day 66

The cold put me completely out of it today; no weights and no cardio, basically the perfect combination to get absolutely no results. With this being the last week before Christmas and I don't see the scale moving much beyond 235, I might be in the ballpark of almost being willing to accept this. My scale needed a new battery (that happens when you put yourself on it on a daily basis) so I replaced the battery but forgot to reset it (it is one of those complicated ones that was the only one I could find that went over three hundred pounds). So when I got on to test it after the battery change it said 116 pounds. In fact when anyone got on it, the thing said 116 pounds. I actually thought of leaving it that way; hey who wouldn't want to be 116 pounds, right? But in the interest of accuracy and, in light of the reality that even my cremated remains would weigh more than 116 pounds, I fixed it so it gave the accurate weight. I can't help but think I will miss seeing 116; maybe I will occasionally pop out that battery just for kicks.

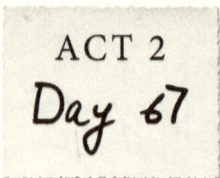

ACT 2

Day 67

All I managed to get in today was some weight training. I have to admit I am starting to enjoy the effects of weight training; I like to see the increasingly noticeable muscles even though I suffer through the process. Hopefully I become one of those people addicted to working out, or at best maybe I can convince myself the pain of the process is worth going through to get the results. Weight training is an interesting undertaking; as soon as you get beyond the basics and look for more options you discover a world of endless information that makes figuring out what to do more difficult than the working out. Luckily I was able to find a few resources for relatively easily understandable additions to my routine. Finding these few gems was one heck of a research project; I think I passed the Holy Grail on my way to useable information.

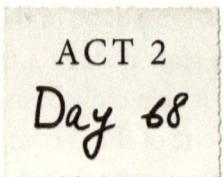

ACT 2

Day 68

Well less than a week to go and, based on my lack of activity today and poor diet, I can assure you that I won't be seeing a number under 235 come Christmas. By poor diet I mean some crackers for my upset stomach and a few pieces of dark chocolate, but I also didn't make sure I ate every couple hours and didn't do any exercise so I know not to expect results. I did find time to research at-home cardio equipment; there are a lot of options in a wide price range. You can spend anywhere from two hundred bucks to over five grand. I am leaning toward just getting a basic stationary bike, that way I can do something a little different that I do when I can get outside.

ACT 2
Day 69

Another Sunday, lazy Sunday. Of course the cold weather and the fact that my back is out gave me a couple A-plus excuses for not doing a damn thing, which means I don't expect a good number on the scale tomorrow. It is so easy to fall off the "exercise and healthy eating" train. The three decades-plus of training has made eating poorly and a sloth-like lifestyle seem second nature. I can feel myself in the center of a dieter's dilemma: I have lost enough weight to look significantly different and the work required to achieve additional smaller and slower results just doesn't seem worth the effort required. Of course if I don't get back on track soon I will be seeing three hundred pounds in no time, so maintaining where I am might have to be motivation enough on most days as the slow process of shedding that last twenty pounds drags on.

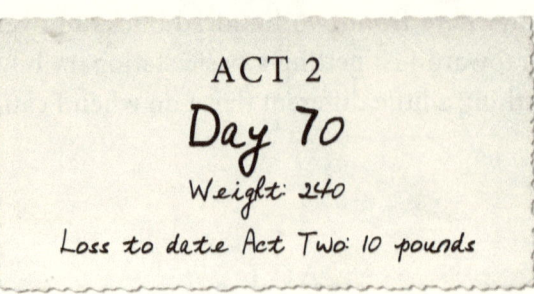

ACT 2

Day 70

Weight: 240

Loss to date Act Two: 10 pounds

Crap. Yeah, that's about all I have to say here: crap. I didn't expect to see such a high number in one week; it feels a lot better to drop five pounds in a week than it does to put on five pounds in a week. What did I do so wrong? Well, let's start with carbohydrates; no matter what I weigh carbohydrates aren't my friend. A few crackers, some white bread, some chips, and a few handfuls of chocolate and watch the scale fly. What else did I do wrong? The lack of exercise didn't compliment my week of carb loading. In my readings I came across this theory that your body has set weights, basically a weight where it is comfortable and from which it resists moving. This makes sense to me, especially how comfortable my body seems at two hundred and forty pounds. It helps explain why all of us trying to lose weight find ourselves struggling to get through various plateaus.

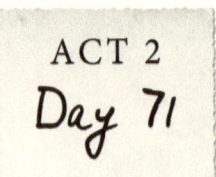

ACT 2

Day 71

I decided Christmas is coming early this year, or, more accurately, my Christmas diet hiatus is coming early. The uphill climb of trying to stick to a strict diet combined with the minuscule weight loss I can expect over the next handful of days has prompted me to fold the diet tent for this year. All in all I would say it was a successful eight months; I am at 240 so I have dropped and kept off sixty-eight pounds but for the most part I would consider Act Two a failure, as the results were not worth the effects of the diet. If you are going to live mainly on bars and shakes do yourself a favor and take advantage of the millions someone else spent on research and development and use one of the prepackaged plans; it is a lot easier to follow. My plan going in is to take three weeks off, but we will see how I feel and how rapidly I expand before deciding whether to cut those three weeks short or not. See you in the New Year!

CHAPTER FIVE

LESSONS LEARNED FROM ACT TWO

Act Two was an eye-opener for this rookie dieter in a lot of ways. First, I would say a highly restrictive diet is not the way I want to continue this journey. In the beginning the results made the suffering worth it but at this point I want real food. Who would want to live on bars and shakes to lose half a pound per week? Not me. Real food is going to be the key to Act Three; that way I can develop a dietary plan that I can live on for the rest of my life that allows for the occasional beak when I really need those high-pleasure foods.

Another important lesson I got out of Act Two is the importance of writing down everything I eat. Without tracking the input there really is no way to know if the results you are seeing are fixable. If there were Ten Commandments of weight loss, tracking your daily input would make the top five for sure.

Act Two also taught me the importance of portion control. Portion size is one of the biggest reasons all the prepared meal plans work: they limit the amount of food you are eating at any given time. We always hear that your stomach is the size of your fist (lucky for me I have big hands) and that the amount of food we take in should not exceed that size. Portion control is a tough one because retraining your brain is a lot harder than training your body, and it hurts a lot more, too.

Lastly, in the post-Act Two landscape it is clear that regular exercise is very important. My thought is that doing a half hour of cardio daily is better than doing an hour every three days. I know a lot of science talks about the "ideal burn zone" but I am less concerned with "ideal burn zone" than with giving my metabolism a daily spike and being able to keep on a program and it is always easier to find a half hour to workout out that it is to find a full hour.

HIATUS TWO

I thought I might cut this short of the originally scheduled three weeks and, what do you know, I have ended it after twelve days. What would prompt such a decision? Well I could easily see that I was recklessly eating again, and the results of that were starting to show up in the lack of room in my pants. It amazes me how quickly I got right back into the "stupid eating" swing: going a long time between meals, eating a ton of carbohydrates, eating late at night; I had it all covered in those twelve days. At least I was smart enough to recognize the problem this time and cut the hiatus short, so, while I might be a slow learner, at least I am learning.

CHAPTER SIX

ACT THREE

GAME PLAN ACT THREE

So now for the real fun: Act Three, living on real foods and still losing weight, also known as "mission impossible." Can a lifetime bad eater find the ability to control his cravings and appetite and discover food combinations that both taste great and are good for you? The game plan going in is simple, because keeping it simple is another thing that would easily make the Ten Commandments of weight loss. My diet will consist of high protein and low carbohydrate combinations and eating every two to three hours, all of which I will track. As far as exercise, after the first week back I plan on doing at least a half hour of cardio every day and weight training three days a week. I will use bars and shakes as meal replacements from time to time but I won't be living on them—thank God.

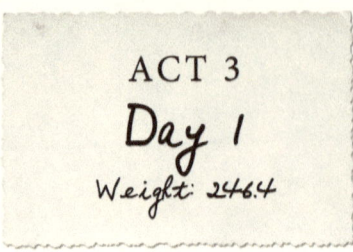

ACT 3
Day 1
Weight: 246.4

Well I was right: the weight was going up. Six and a half pounds gained in twelve days; now that's impressive. Maybe I can write a weight-gaining book for skinny folks, because I have weight gaining down to a science. Today was simple; I ate less than 1500 high protein, low carbohydrate calories, drank enough water, and made sure I had my meals every two to three hours. The pounds should start falling off, right? Oddly enough as I start this sensible eating act, life happened and we have to go to Michigan for a funeral at the end of this week. This will be an ideal time to begin my experiment about finding a healthy way to eat out. The big thing for me is to not let this be an ex-cuse to fall—or more accurately waddle—off the wagon. My goal this week is simple: at the end of this week I want to be in the 243-range and to do this I can't go off track just because I am away from home. I did make sure to book a hotel with a fitness center, so I can get my indoor cardio in, and I have my notebook ready to track what I take in. The sooner I get back under 240 the better, though; I liked the look and feel of the high 230s a lot more than I do the mid-240s, which seems odd to me since it is less than ten pounds—but trust me, those few pounds do make a big difference.

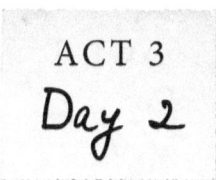

ACT 3

Day 2

Day two is always a tough day on the diet train. I know that if I make it past day three it will get a lot easier until those late-teen days, but that knowledge doesn't make day two any easier. Now that it's the beginning of a new year the endless parade of "lose weight quick and easy" commercials are out in full force. There are actually a few that are realistic, both in their weight-loss promises and their choice of pitch people, which is refreshing. The reality is we won't all look like those perfect models who have the benefit of years of exercising and healthy eating combined with genetics, but we can all improve on where we are. At some point we need to get to a position where we measure health improvement, rather than living by the scale and seeking some ideal.

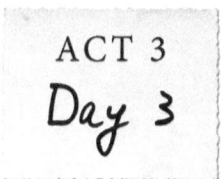

ACT 3

Day 3

Today I managed to fight off the urge to jump on the scale; I plan on giving the diet one more day before risking seeing a number that would send me over the edge. Wow do I need to get over my scale obsession. So again life happened and I have a toothache; nothing major but enough to make eating less appealing. Hey, maybe I discovered a new diet success secret: tooth pain to a thinner you. Sadly I will have to get it fixed once I get back into town, so it won't be a long-lasting diet solution.

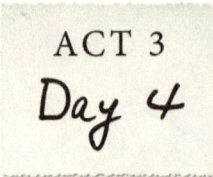

ACT 3

Day 4

Some days the scale just makes you smile & today was one of those days: 239.2. If I can weigh the same when I get back from my trip to Michigan on Tuesday I will consider this a success to date. It is amazing how quickly the weight comes off in the first few days, but it did go on really quickly once I went off the diet. Maybe my body is adjusting to the idea that its normal weight is in the high 230s; one can hope. Did some more thinking of how to move away from relying solely on the scale to gauge my success, and I came up with something fairly simple. Since there are few things simpler than getting dressed, I figured why not use clothes size as well as weight and measurements. With that in mind, I am going to focus on getting my weight under 220 pounds, my suit size to a 42 long (right now I am a 44 long), my shirt size to a large, and my pants size to a size 34 (right now I am a 36; remember I started at a size 44!).

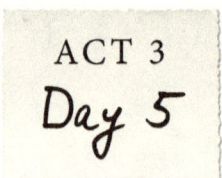

ACT 3

Day 5

There is nothing like an airport to promote unhealthy eating. I was actually good through the airport experience; luckily I remembered to bring some bars with me so I was able to resist the temptation of the airport food court, which the boredom of being in an airport always magnifies. Dinner once we got into town was even easier;

we went somewhere where I could get chicken fajitas, can't really go wrong there. One day down, three to go.

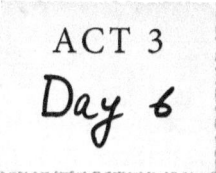

ACT 3
Day 6

Today was the funeral, and I must say the menu at the reception that followed offered very little temptation. The really only bad thing I ate was a small amount of cake. However, afterward I didn't do as well; seems the temptation of gas station offerings combined with the boredom of being buried in snow combined with the feelings a funeral brings to the table was too much. I ate more carbohydrates today than I have in the past five days, topped off with pizza for dinner, because hey, we are in a hotel in a town buried in snow. What are we supposed to order? Hopefully tomorrow will go better.

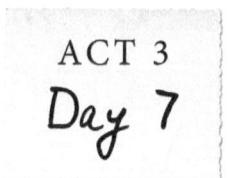

ACT 3
Day 7

I have to get home before I have to buy bigger pants. Today was the worst eating day to date: another round of gas station munchies and a second helping of pizza. I am sure I have put on two to three pounds already. We fly home tomorrow; hopefully I can manage to survive and get myself back on track before I undo all my hard work. Clearly it is going to take me a while to figure out how to successfully maintain a sensible diet while traveling.

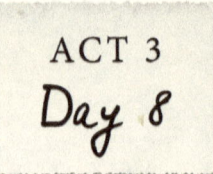

ACT 3
Day 8

On the upside, traveling back home today means I don't have to get on the scale, which is a good thing considering how poorly I ate the last four days. There is a way to maintain a sensible diet when you are traveling, but I assure you I have not found it. If anything, a trip out of town becomes a food orgy for me. I really need to fix that out or just stop leaving town. Well, made it home in one piece, ate horribly, and tomorrow I get to jump on the scale. Wish me luck.

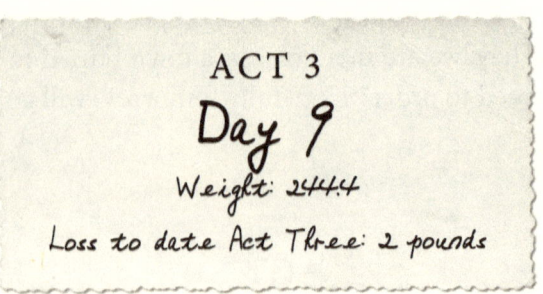

ACT 3
Day 9
Weight: 244.4
Loss to date Act Three: 2 pounds

So four good days and four bad days and I lost two pounds. I am going to call that a win. I mean, why not? It's not like calling it a loss would change the results, right? Today was a good diet day: ate every couple hours, drank a good amount of water, and kept the calorie count under 1500. However, as it got later in the evening I seemed to get hungrier and hungrier, it's amazing how quickly my body remembers the joys of late-night gorging. It probably didn't help that I spent the past four days gorging late at night.

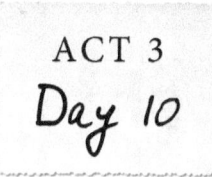

ACT 3
Day 10

Second day back on the plan and, as usual, the first few days really suck. The toughest struggle is always in the beginning; after a few days you do get used to it, I promise. I kept the calories under 1500 for the second day in a row so I expect some serious results. Today was a long, long workday but I still managed to keep my calorie count in line. I read a bunch of health and fitness articles today, always a good way to keep you on a diet, and I must say there is a lot of garbage out there. This stuff isn't as complicated as people asking for your credit card number make it out to be. The reality is that weight loss is nothing more than burning more calories than you take in, eating the right foods, eating small portions every couple hours, and exercising.

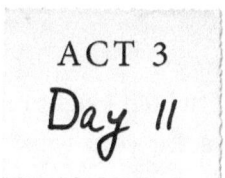

ACT 3
Day 11

Fantastic scale day: 239.4! Thankfully I managed to take off all the weight I put on during our trip to Michigan so I am back on track. Hopefully before my next weight day I can drop another couple pounds. Looking back, I haven't had the scale under 235 so that would be an ideal mark to hit. I don't see that happening in the next three days, though. We made plans to have a friend visit over Super Bowl weekend in three weeks so I better get working on the menu because, like me, he likes his junk food. Better to be prepared than cursing the scale the next day.

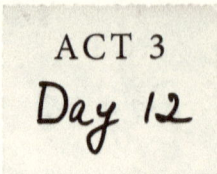

ACT 3

Day 12

Nothing like a trip to the dentist to throw your day off kilter. The problem was no big deal and I was in and out in an hour, which turned out to be the perfect amount of time to ruin my plans for the day. Although I wanted to reward myself with some comfort food—you know pizza, ice cream, cookies, and the like—I controlled myself and stuck to the plan keeping my daily intake under 1500. We will see where it gets us in another couple days.

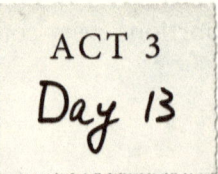

ACT 3

Day 13

Football playoff weekend, which used to mean an endless buffet of the best-tasting and "worst for your waist line" foods the world has to offer. This year is a bit different—okay, a lot different. Today I again kept the intake right around 1500 calories, despite the great games on the TV. It is odd how we so easily attach gorging ourselves to viewing an athletic competition. You would think the sight of such athletic excellence would propel us off the couch and get us to exercise, but nope. Just watch the commercials: an endless parade of calories, followed by an ad for a car to take you to the fast-food provider whose commercial follows.

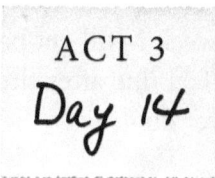

ACT 3

Day 14

Another day of playoff football and another day of keeping the calories under 1500; I'd better see results tomorrow morning! I have adjusted to the new eating routine, or should I say *re*-adjusted, after my four-day feast in Michigan. So far I have kept my dietary selection simply: turkey sandwiches on sourdough bread, chicken—lots of chicken, including homemade barbeque chicken pizza—Jell-O with fruit, occasional helpings of unsalted peanuts, and protein bars and shakes. I am planning on switching to whole grain and rye breads, since I have recently read a couple reports that said rye bread keeps you full longer and whole grain can help to reduce that stubborn abdominal fat—I can use all the help there I can get.

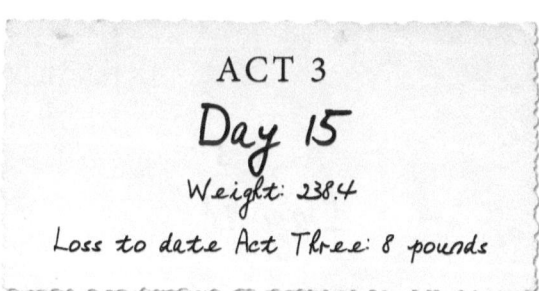

ACT 3

Day 15

Weight: 238.4

Loss to date Act Three: 8 pounds

I was expecting the scale to still be above 239, so I couldn't have been happier this morning. This puts me at exactly seventy pounds lost. I set a short-term goal: sub-235 by Super Bowl weekend, which is three weeks from yesterday. I got back to walking today; only did two miles, which is usually where I have been starting after my breaks from working out. My plan is to do two miles four days this week, then increase it weekly by six-tenths of a mile until I am at five miles. Starting next week I will get back to the weights on the three non-cardio days. I feel fine after the two miles, worked up a good sweat and, didn't over do it.

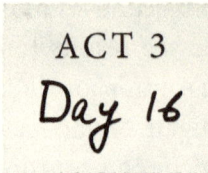

ACT 3
Day 16

I may have spoken to soon when I said I didn't hurt myself with yesterday's two-mile walk. All last night I kept waking up with pain in my knee; not a pleasant way to sleep. Outside of that I am fine so hopefully it is just a temporary issue. I had a business dinner tonight and really did pretty well considering the wealth of calorie-packed options on the menu, sticking with a basic chicken sandwich. Hopefully my restraint pays off.

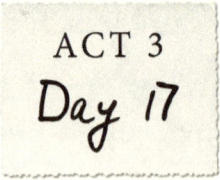

ACT 3
Day 17

Our scale broke so we had to get a new one and it read 238.8. While that .4 pounds could be a difference in the two scales, I really am not concerned with it: 238 is 238. If the weight keeps coming off and I can steadily increase my walking distance weekly I should be in real good shape to try a 10K. Nice how it all works out in theory; now to make it work in practice!

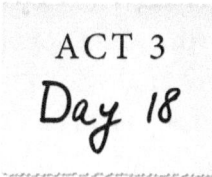

ACT 3
Day 18

I had little to no pain today so maybe I am adjusting to the walking again quickly. Had to pick up new sneakers; let me warn you expect to go through sneakers every three to six months if you are walking a lot. I am not one for expensive sneakers; the ones I bought today were under fifty bucks. They are a different brand than my usual so we will see how they work out. We made a great turkey chili tonight, which was perfect given the chill in the air. It is a really basic recipe: ground turkey, three types of beans, chicken broth, and tomato sauce. I didn't do an accurate calorie count but come on, how many calories could be in all that lean protein? Now I did have three bowls of it, and you know nothing goes better with chili than fresh sourdough bread so I might have splurged a bit but compared to how I used to splurge this should be no problem. Besides I am not getting back on the scale till Monday, and as long as I have dropped more than one and a half pounds it's yet another victory week!

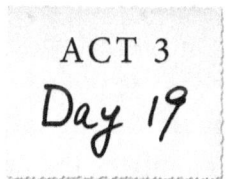

ACT 3
Day 19

Breaking in new shoes is never a pleasant experience. This new brand is a little more snug, which I hoped would correct my walking since now I know there is a proper way to walk to reduce knee and ankle pain. From what I learned in my two miles today, as long

I walk with proper form—heal hitting first—the shoes are fine, but when I walk the way I have been for however long I've been walking, which is basically the whole foot flopping to the ground at once, then I get a pain in my right ankle. So in theory, at least these shoes should force me to correct my form and save me some knee pain, assuming relearning to walk doesn't kill me in the process. Today was another good diet day: still keeping the calories at around 1500, so hopefully the weight will continue to fall off. I need to figure out more real food options on this program. Typically I have been eating three protein bars a day and, while they are low in calories and carbohydrates as well as high in protein, they are also harder for my system to digest. My body would appreciate more real food and fewer of those processed bars.

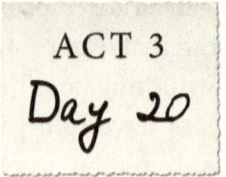

ACT 3

Day 20

Another good diet day, but some of the information I have been reading has me wondering if what I am eating really is good for me. To keep the science to a minimum: there are factors in processed food, pesticides used on produce and fruits, plastic packaging used in foods, as well as other sources that basically screw with your hormone levels and tell your body to put on and keep fat. New studies and reports appear all the time trying to answer the fat question; there is even the idea of identifying the "fat gene" and trying to reprogram it. Some of this is science fiction and some of it serves no other purpose than marketing a product but this particular research actually makes sense. Look at how our eating has changed as people: basically we got further away from the source of our food and replaced pure food with prepackaged and processed food. As we have done that, we have gotten more and more obese. Going forward I need to design this program around pure foods and fewer processed foods. This will be tough because I have become accustomed to relying on protein bars, but if I could get use to eating protein bars I am sure I can make this adjustment too.

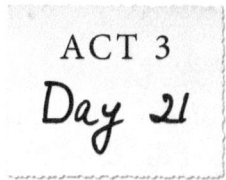

ACT 3
Day 21

Weather did not cooperate with my plans to get some cardio in, but I still should be in the 237s tomorrow, which keeps me on track to hit 225 in about nine weeks. While this week may not have a huge loss, I have to look at the fact that I dropped over six pounds in three weeks. Speaking of regular healthy diets, I looked back on my daily eating and found I tend to eat two regular meals and three or four bars a day. As my first step toward eating more "pure" foods, I am going to switch that to two bars and three regular meals a day. When I eat regular food I do eat really pure, grilled chicken without any sauces or creams, whole grain beads, smoked turkey, eggs, beans, and the like, so I should make the transition easily; hopefully I can keep the weight coming off through the transition. Avoiding the pesticides and plastic-wrapped foods will be much tougher, though.

ACT 3
Day 22
Weight: 238.4
Loss to date Act Three: 8 pounds

So I lost zero pounds in the last week; pretty pathetic in itself, but I had to expect that, since I did drop six pounds in the past three weeks. Hopefully this week I will have some positive movement on the scale. I am mixing it up this week, introducing more foods to the mix including salads and more fruits and vegetables. Needless to say figuring all this out will be complicated and involve trial and error (hopefully not too much error). To start with, I am limiting myself to two protein bars a day, which should help with the upset stomach I have been suffering, and instead taking more calories in from pure sources like whole grain bread, lean protein (turkey, chicken, eggs, and beans), green vegetables, and fruits.

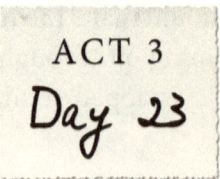

ACT 3
Day 23

Made it through a very long and stressful day today without going over 1500 calories! It might not sound like much to some but to someone who has spent his entire adult life turning to the fridge for therapy that is huge. I picked up some organic chicken for dinner, and let me tell you: expect to pay about twice as much, but also expect it to taste twice as good. Since I eat so little food I figured I might as well eat the very best.

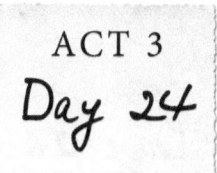

ACT 3

Day 24

Made it through the day with only one bar; it is nice when you make enough time in the morning to make breakfast (for me it was a two-egg omelet over a piece of whole grain toast total: calories, 260) so you don't start your day with a food supplement but rather real food. Speaking of calories, mine crept up to about 1700 today, but since I had five meals of real food I can live with that. Got another 2.6 miles in today so let's see what kind of results we have for tomorrow's midweek weigh-in! Any guesses? I'm going with 237 because I deserve a pound plus off after doing a net-zero last week.

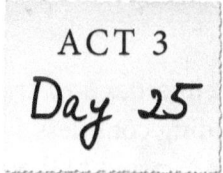

ACT 3

Day 25

Success on the scale today: 236.8! Not a lot of protein bars or shakes this week, which makes the weight drop even better. What could be better than eating regular foods and losing weight? Took it easy today; I have had a stomach issue for the last week. Remember, stomach issues were what got me on this program in the first place, which is why I still say the bad news was that it wasn't a heart attack. A heart attack, assuming you survive that is, is a onetime event:

change your diet a bit, lose some weight, take some pills, and get back at it. With a stomach disorder it's more like change your diet, drop a ton of weight, and realize the problem will keep coming back.

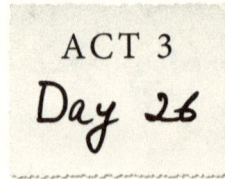

ACT 3

Day 26

Another day partially sidelined with a stomach issue. I did manage to get my walking in but suffered through it and could tell I was moving slower. But hey, I still got it in. I will have to suffer through it since I don't want to live the rest of my life on pills.

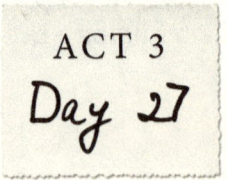

ACT 3

Day 27

Another day with stomach issues so I tried to take it easy. I have spent countless hours reading countless articles online about stomach issues since this thing started bothering me about two weeks ago. The beauty of the Internet is also its greatest drawback: endless information. The best I can hope for is this to pass quickly, but regardless I plan on living my life and doing what I need to do to keep my fitness bus rolling.

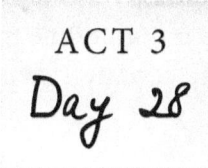

ACT 3

Day 28

Yet another day spent trying to get over my stomach issues. If someone else was suffering like this for this long the first thing I would say is, "Get to a doctor." But for me this isn't something new, and I have a family history of stomach problems so I have a pretty good idea what the problem is and plan wait it out. Tomorrow is another weigh day and I am not expecting much since my activity has been restricted and I have been using crackers to ease my stomach pains. Right now I am not overly concerned about what the scale says—actually, scratch that. I don't really care what it says. Hopefully I can get back to exercising soon.

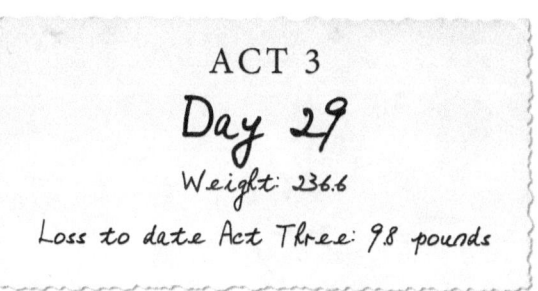

ACT 3

Day 29

Weight: 236.6

Loss to date Act Three: 9.8 pounds

So four weeks in and I have lost almost ten pounds. I am still suffering with a stomach issue, so I decided to take this week off from walking; we are having a friend in visit at the end of this week for four days so I want to be as close to over this stomach issue as possible by then so we can properly show him the town. My goal for this time next week is to still weigh in the 236-range, since I will have company and that typically involves poor eating. If I start next week at the same weight I am today, I will consider that a victory. This week also marks the ninth month of me trying to lose weight; nine months and I have dropped seventy-two pounds—not too shabby.

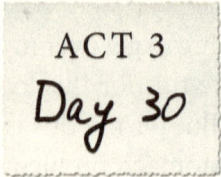

ACT 3

Day 30

So I decided to take the whole day off today, and tried to rest in the hopes of my stomach recovering in time for the weekend. Let's hope it works. It seems weird to suffer from stomach issues considering I don't really eat much that would cause that to happen. I guess that's the magic of genetics. Today I read that a high protein diet can cause stomach issues to flare up, so maybe that's it. Who knows at this point; I just want it to go away so I can get back to my regular diet and exercise routine.

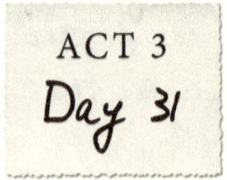

ACT 3

Day 31

Today I felt somewhat better so I did manage to get out and get some work done. Also found a 5K that occurs right around the one-year anniversary of my fitness quest; sounds like a sign from God doesn't it? Maybe I will skip the 10K (especially since I first noticed the stomach issues when I was walking) and instead do the 5K, which I know I can handle. I don't want to do the type of damage to myself that requires any long recovery periods, and I have enough potential injury spots that being careful is very important.

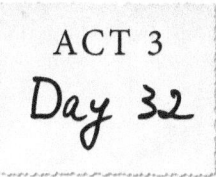

ACT 3

Day 32

Feeling closer to human today, thankfully. Maybe this program has taught me to learn to listen to my body, at least occasionally. Still keeping the calories in line, no more than 1500 a day, but haven't started exercising again yet. I braved the scale today: 236.4. At least I haven't gained any weight being ill and rooted to my couch. Hopefully I can continue that through the weekend and start fresh losing pounds come Monday.

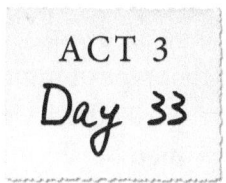

ACT 3

Day 33

Feeling much better today and can't wait to be back to one hundred percent. We got hit by a massive rainstorm today, which reminded me I still have to get indoor cardio equipment. I am considering getting a punching bag so I can add something interesting to the routine, since diversity is important to maintaining a training program. Besides when you're denying yourself food, and you love food, you do run across the desire to hit something every so often. Based on my own subjective scale I would say I started out obese and, after nine months, I have achieved a doughy physique. Sure, I could lament on how I am still a doughboy, but I look a lot better than I did as a beached whale. You have to focus on the progress. This is another reason to keep the old fat clothes and old photos of the fatter you handy: to see how far you have come. In the next couple weeks, once I know I can get back to working out, I will take measurements again and see how far I have come and try to figure out where I want to be.

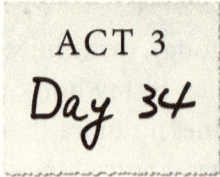

ACT 3

Day 34

The stomach is getting better by the day. I really think the probiotics and green tea I have been enjoying are helping. I spoke to a friend today who is again back in the weight loss battle and he just spent a couple grand on equipment. Not that there is anything wrong with buying workout equipment, but based on his track record in a few weeks that equipment will be an overpriced clothes hamper. Some people argue that putting that type of money out will help force you to work out, but if that were true there wouldn't be so many obese people with monthly gym memberships fees being sucked out of their checking accounts.

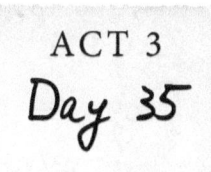

ACT 3
Day 35

Super Bowl Sunday: every year up until this one this was a day to feast until it hurt, then rest, then feast some more. Today obviously was a bit different. We had our patent-worthy homemade barbeque chicken pizza, and as a snack I had grapes and carrots with light ranch dressing. Our family friend had to cancel his planned visit; maybe the menu scared him off. Had you asked me any year before this one I would have told you these weren't Super Bowl-worthy eats, but this year it was just right. Taking those first three months and eating nothing but the program bars and shakes did wonders for me; it allowed me to reset my body and, more importantly, my mind, so my thoughts on food have changed. When you go three months without any normal foods your whole idea of what normal food is actually changes. You can think of what you are eating rather than shoving whatever sounds good into your face. I know it sounds strange, and believe me nine months ago I wouldn't have believed it myself. Tomorrow is a weight day; five weeks into Act Three. Let's hope progress is still being made.

ACT 3

Day 36

Weight: 237.6

Loss to date Act Three: 8.8 pounds

Well at least the week wasn't too bad. Losing a week to the couch and crackers by the mouthful, I expected much worse results. Time to get back on track and the best place to start is diet. Since my stomach isn't one hundred percent yet I am still hesitant about exercising.

ACT 3

Day 37

Wow, was that a busy day. I am catching up on the work I missed the past few days. Based on the amount of stuff I produced today I should have dropped a couple pounds easily, so I figure I will check tomorrow morning and see.

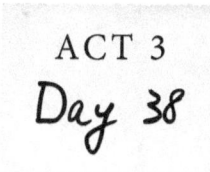

ACT 3
Day 38

Well it worked: I was 235 this morning! This is a number I haven't seen in a while; in fact I was beginning to doubt if my scale actually went that low. I guess office work can be a good weight loss workout. Or maybe it is because for the past two days I have been very diligently tracking everything I eat and not allowing myself to use an unhappy stomach to justify shoving crackers down my throat. Yeah, I would have to say it's controlling the intake of food rather than my work output that made the difference. My goal for the rest of the week is to get under 235. I don't care if that means the scale says 234.9 next Monday; anything under 235 is a win for this week.

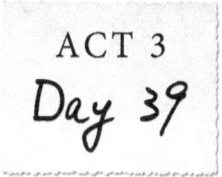

ACT 3
Day 39

Well I made it through another busy day without breaking the 1500-calorie limit. I can tell you firsthand: once you give yourself enough time to adapt to a restricted calorie diet it becomes easier and easier to stick within that limit. Still not working out yet and I am beginning to miss it—or, let me be more accurate: my body is beginning to miss it. Long work days spend hunched over a computer are rough on the back, and my back can attest to the fact that I have put some long days in lately, so hopefully next week I can get back to working out.

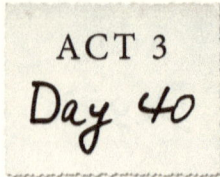

ACT 3

Day 40

It is a good thing I am not walking because we got snow for the first time in a decade where I live. How many more signs do I need to see before making an investment in indoor cardio equipment? Like most people, when I was trapped inside I had to fight the temptation to overeat. Luckily I had plenty of work to keep me busy (never thought I would consider myself lucky to have plenty of work to do). So I would say I was successful at keeping my calories below the 1500-calorie mark.

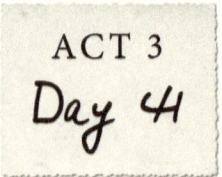

ACT 3

Day 41

Today was the day before Valentine's Day so I braved what snow managed to stick and went to the store. I would love to tell you I stuck with just flowers but I also picked up some chocolate. I was smart enough to stick to dark chocolate without any filling so the pieces I eat—and if there is chocolate in the house I am eating it—shouldn't cause me too much harm. Besides, it is Valentine's Day; you have to live a little bit. I have put in a lot of time reading about the benefits of green tea; let me tell you go get yourself some green tea! I first began taking it for my stomach and it seemed to help but it also is supposed to be good for weight loss (both the caffeine and catechins in green tea help with weight loss), prevention and treatment of cancer, helping lower cholesterol, and a host of other things. There are questions about how accurate these findings are but I can tell you it has helped my stomach and I plan to keep taking it since it is so much easier on my stomach than coffee. If I can get an added weight loss benefit that's a bonus.

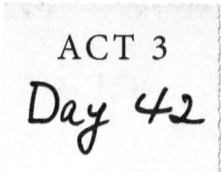

ACT 3

Day 42

Valentine's Day: nothing says "I love you" like a fistful of empty calories. Hopefully I didn't do too much scale damage, but either way if you can't occasionally enjoy life what is the point?

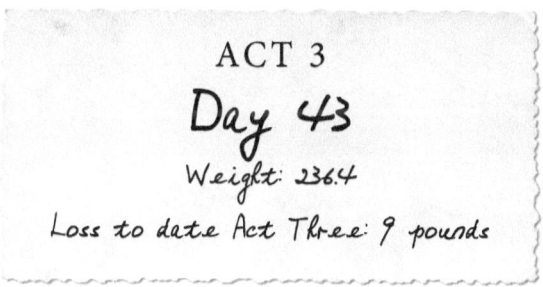

ACT 3

Day 43

Weight: 236.4

Loss to date Act Three: 9 pounds

Well I didn't finish the week under 235 but hey, I did drop over a pound this week despite battling Valentine's Day. This week my goal is to get the diet back under 1500 calories a day, drink at least 100 ounces of water a week, and drink two cups of green tea a day. I also expect to be able to start working out at the end of this week; I am targeting Friday as my restart date. I figure if I can do all those things I should have no problem being under 235 in seven days. This will be a busy workweek so hopefully I can keep myself on track. Looking at the weight loss so far—eight pounds in six weeks—it doesn't sound overly impressive but remember it is more than a pound a week and I am eating normal food, not exercising and even managed to enjoy chocolate and a weekend of poor eating while out of town. All things considered, not bad results.

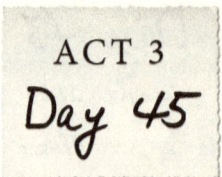

ACT 3

Day 44

I lost another day to an irritated stomach; at some point I might give up and go to the doctor. Hopefully I can find a way to balance out my unhappy stomach without dedicating a hundred dollars a month to pills that just mask the problem. We will see.

ACT 3

Day 45

It is amazing how long a bag or two of chocolate lasts when you are trying to watch your caloric intake. I don't know if I would be better off stuffing my face with all the chocolate in one day and getting back on the diet track or not, but we still have some and I can't help myself but to eat a handful a couple times a day. These little treats aren't making it onto my food-tracking sheet, but I can estimate that I am eating about ten pieces a day three different times, which is about 400 extra calories. When I went to the grocery today

I skipped the chocolate and got some unsalted peanuts and crackers to snack on (peanuts are a good source of protein and the crackers help ease my stomach woes). We had turkey burgers for the first time tonight made with fresh-ground turkey; they basically are just like a hamburger in that they taste like whatever you put on them (mustard, relish, and onion for me) with the exception that they cook to a different color (light brown). I have had people try to feed me these things in the past and I thought they were slimy and simply wrong, but if you use fresh-ground turkey they are actually pretty good–and obviously much better for you than beef. So now we have a little more variety in our dining options thanks to my wife bravely putting a turkey burger in front of me.

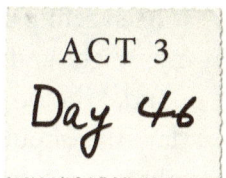

ACT 3
Day 46

Today was Thursday, which is our official day off around here. Since we both are self-employed and tend to work on the weekends, we decided to take Thursdays off to spend together. Today we went downtown and wandered the streets like two wide-eyed tourists. After a couple hours of walking we decided to brave a restaurant and get something to eat. We went to one of our favorite places and I had a buffalo chicken cheesesteak and sweet potato fries. There are more calories in this one meal than I have been eating a day, and I ordered this fully assuming my stomach would react in a rather unhappy matter. Well, to the contrary, I actually had no negative response to the meal at all. We spent another couple hours afterward wandering around and I had no issues with my stomach; in fact, I would say my stomach actually felt the closest to normal as it has in a few weeks. This got me thinking that maybe my diet might be causing some of the stomach issues after all. Time to do some research and experimenting; this should be fun.

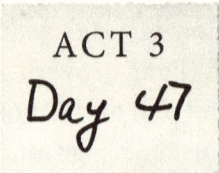

ACT 3

Day 47

I did some research and it turns out my body needs 3700 calories a day to function, which means it takes 3700 calories a day to maintain my current weight. Since I have been limiting it to around 1500 calories I shouldn't be shocked that my stomach, which has a history of issues with high acid levels, has been acting up. So if I need to eat 3700 calories a day to maintain my weight and it takes a deficit of 3500 calories a week to lose one pound, I should be able to drop a pound a week eating 3000 calories a day. This should be enough in theory to ease my stomach woes. It might take a couple weeks for my stomach and body to get back to normal and adjust to this new higher daily calorie limit so I am expecting to gain a couple pounds over the next couple weeks. From now on I have to stop focusing on the scale and start focusing on my health and listening to my body. The scale can be a good tool up until a point but then if you obsess about a stupid number on a stupid piece of machinery you start doing stupid things to your body when your whole intent was to get healthier.

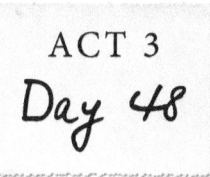

ACT 3
Day 48

Two days of eating regular food at about 2300 calories a day and I already feel better. Really makes me wonder if I brought my stomach issues on myself. I mean you hear of that happening to teenage girls with eating problems but come on: I am almost forty and still so fat it couldn't happen to me. Well, maybe it did. I guess time will tell. So I discovered there really are four pillars to health for those of us over thirty: nutrition (which I am still trying to figure out), strength-training (which I begin again next week), cardiovascular exercise (again beginning next week), and flexibility training (I still have to research exactly what that means). As it turns out, as we age our muscles get stiffer and stiffer and we increase our odds of hurting ourselves doing normal things because of this increased stiffness, so we must work to improve our flexibility, which I will get right on as soon as I know exactly what that actually means.

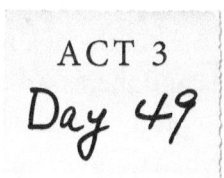

ACT 3
Day 49

Another day of eating regular foods and another day of decreased stomach pains; it looks like I might have solved the problem–or actually been the problem in the first place. Tomorrow when I weigh-in I will also be doing all the measurements I did when I began so I can see how far I have come. For cardio it is back to walking, starting at two miles and working it up from there, just like starting all over again.

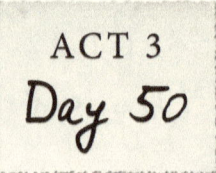

ACT 3
Day 50

MEASUREMENTS

	Start	Now	Change
Weight:	308.4	238	-70.4 pounds
Chest:	47	42	-5 inches
Waist:	46.5	39	-7.5 inches
Abs:	49	40	-9 inches
Arms:	14.5	13.5	-1 inch
Thigh:	27.25	22	-5.25 inches

There is no way I can complain about this type of success. Sure my weight is up, but only by two tenths of a pound since Friday when I switched to all real foods and increased my calories from 1500 to close to 2500. I probably should have done measurements all along to track my progress; maybe taking them once a month, but there is a certain satisfaction in seeing such a large change at one time. More of my focus will be on toning and shaping what I have, hoping more fat comes off and more muscle comes on. My plan was to start working out today but I had to visit my doctor to deal with a staph infection so I am going to start tomorrow. On the plus side, I found a good doctor who I will be working with going forward, starting with dealing with my recurring stomach issues. Like I have said before, life does happen as you try to get yourself in better shape so you have to be able to adjust. Spending two hours in the doctor's office and the effects of the antibiotics were enough to get me to put off working out; besides I still have to figure out exactly what flexibility training is. My plan is to get my walk in early in the morning then get my workday in and do the weight training at night. From what I read, that is considered ideal if you are doing both cardio and weight training on the same day so we will see how it works. Time to go figure out what flexibility training is.

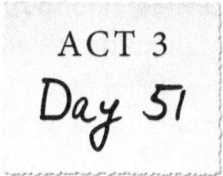

ACT 3
Day 51

Talk about being thrown a curve ball. The antibiotics I am taking wrecked me, and any plans I had to get back to working out. Funny—the side effects of the antibiotics turned out to be worse than the problem the antibiotics were supposed to address. I barely made it through my day. On the plus side I did manage to successfully navigate a lunch menu for a business meeting that didn't feature smart eating or low calorie options. I kept it simple: grilled chicken and mashed potatoes. Heading back in to the doctor tomorrow to hopefully get this antibiotic changed.

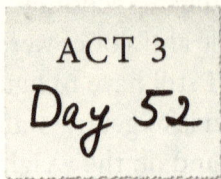

ACT 3

Day 52

At least I am developing a good working relationship with my primary care physician, seeing how I have seen her twice in three days. It turns out that I have shingles, which is basically adult chicken pox brought on by a weakened immune system (geez, think that maybe suffering with a bad stomach for a month before I changed my diet could have weakened my immune system?). So after suffering to sleep last night because of a literal pain in my neck, I have new antibiotics, painkillers, and about three weeks before I recover. Hopefully I begin to feel more human soon so I can get back to working out, however slowly.

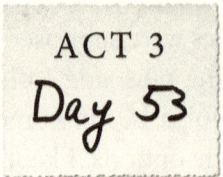

ACT 3

Day 53

Well not much accomplished today: three antibiotics and a painkiller make getting anything done nearly impossible. As part of my healing process I am doing plenty of comfort eating, though, so that should create a scale change although not in the direction I want. I'd better get well quick before I am dressing in the fat clothes closet.

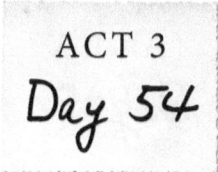

ACT 3

Day 54

All right, feeling a bit better today; about fifty percent human I would say. My hope is to be about seventy-five percent by Monday so I can get back to my life, at least seventy-five percent of it. Assuming I feel better I will be getting my diet back on track next week and begin working out slowly. It sucks to lose a week but I have to get my health back. You just have to love when life happens and derails your otherwise perfect plans, don't you?

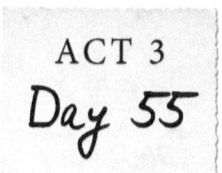

ACT 3

Day 55

This recovery thing is getting way beyond boring. I have been comfort eating like there actually may not be a tomorrow so I should have an awesome number on the scale in a couple days. My hope is if I really rest—I mean really, really rest as in do nothing—for a couple days I will feel much better and be able to get at it again.

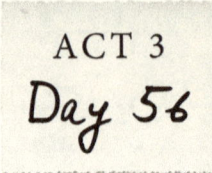

ACT 3

Day 56

Today was another do nothing recovery day. I did look into flexibility training; turns out it's yoga, who knew. My plan is to start doing some light lifting tomorrow and if all goes as planned I should be mixing in some basic yoga by the end of the week and begin cardio again next week—again assuming everything goes as planned. I also plan on fixing my diet over the next couple weeks and then reducing the calories over the last five to six weeks to slightly less than 2000 a day to hopefully spike the weight loss; we will see if that works.

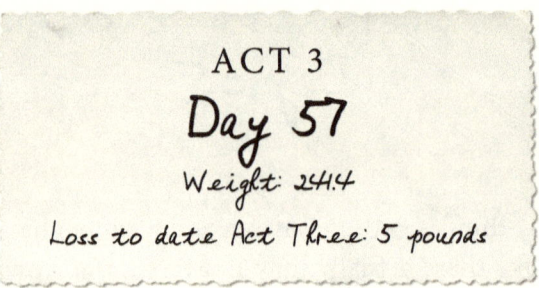

ACT 3

Day 57

Weight: 244.4

Loss to date Act Three: 5 pounds

Well that sucks: fifty-seven days and a net loss of five pounds. I figured the scale would be higher today, seeing how I spent the past five days comfort eating but it still sucks to see that after fifty-seven days I have only lost five pounds. With nine weeks left I really have to get it in gear. Today I did some strength-training, focusing on my lower body since a lot of the research I did the past couple days suggested that one of the best ways to build muscle burning fat is to strength-train your lower body. I found a three-day-a-week strength-training program to do and will combine that with three days a week of flexibility work (sorry, just can't bring myself to say I am doing yoga yet). Starting next week I will be doing four days of cardio as well; that should be a winning combination that burns at least 2000 extra calories a week and, if I combine that with a weekly calorie deficiency of 2400, I should drop 1.25 pound a week; at least that's how the math works out. After working out for the first time in what seems like forever my legs are jelly right now but I am sure I will get use to it at some point. Wish me luck tomorrow when I hit the flexibility-training mat.

ACT 3
Day 58

One day of exercising and wow did I feel it. It does make me think that what I read was right: the best way to build muscle-burning fat is by doing compound movements and working your lower body; my legs feel like they are on fire today, which must mean calories are being burnt. Today I did my flexibility training, nothing too complex, just a handful of very simple positions. I have to admit that it actually made my back feel a lot better. Like a lot of people my job requires me to spend most of the working day on my butt, so my back pays the price. Hopefully this flexibility-training continues to help.

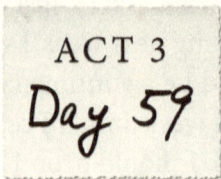

ACT 3

Day 59

Today was upper body weight training day, and boy is my upper body in need of training. Just like the lower body workout, this is a five- to six- exercise routine that focuses on being time efficient and utilizing compound movements. It is amazing how much you can get done in a short period of time when you do the right exercises. I really felt these first two workouts so I expect some decent results in the next couple weeks. My diet has been kept to right around 2500 calories a day; I have been eating every two to three hours, mainly fresh fruits and lean proteins in addition to drinking plenty of water, so we should see some good results in another few days.

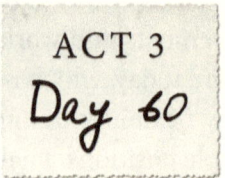

ACT 3

Day 60

I went so long without working out and my body is feeling every bit of it. That is one of the biggest mistakes I have made along this journey: I should have kept working out all along. So my advice is wherever you are on this journey keep working out, even if you have to step it down a bit. Just don't stop because when you restart it will hurt and hurt a lot. I did more yoga today—figured I might as well call it what it is—and again kept my calorie count under 2500. Next week I am throwing cardio into the mix so the weight should be flying off, or at least let's hope it does.

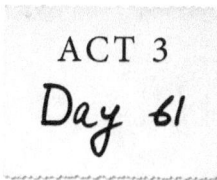

ACT 3

Day 61

Got through the first half of a whole body circuit workout before pulling something in my left calf. See what happens when you go to long without working out? Hopefully if nothing else this book serves as a reminder to keep working out to avoid the pains associated with constantly stopping and starting. So far the daily calories are still under 2500 so I should see some good results on the scale soon.

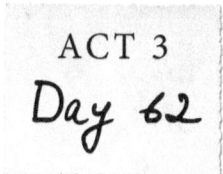

ACT 3

Day 62

No weights today, I did a short walk and took the bulk of the day off. I am really good at putting weight on, if I workout I put on muscle quickly and if I eat poorly I put on pounds quickly. I might have to suffer with a slightly higher number on the scale because of the weight training I am doing, but my wife prefers even the slightest muscle pump I get from working out and that's way more important than a number on a scale.

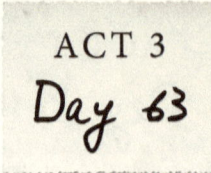

ACT 3

Day 63

I picked up a pull-up bar today, not a great idea. Not that it isn't a great exercise, but there are few things as humiliating as realizing you can't pull yourself up. It is amazing: push-ups I can do no problem, but pull-ups I have no chance of doing right now. It's okay; I will get there, eventually, I hope.

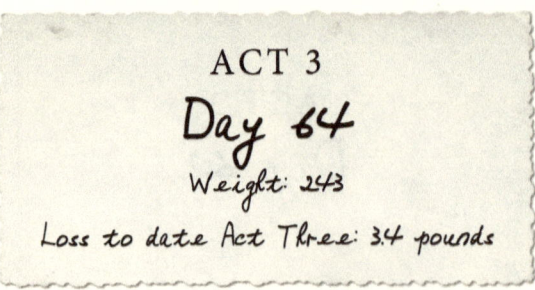

ACT 3

Day 64

Weight: 243

Loss to date Act Three: 34 pounds

Well after a week of eating right, around 2500 calories a day, doing flexibility-training, and three days of strength-training I gained over a pound, lucky me. Now before we hit the panic button this is to be expected for a few reasons. First I am inclined to put weight on quickly, whether its muscle from strength-training or fat from eating poorly. Second, since it has been so long since I did any strength-training my body is adjusting to this new addition to its routine. Third, I did zero cardio last week and I dramatically increased my calories. When you combine those factors you need to expect to see the scale move up a bit. Starting this week I am adding four days of cardio (starting with two miles of walking today) so I expect the scale to move down over the next couple weeks. Much more importantly, my body is looking a lot better (much better than it looked when I was eight pounds lighter) and my clothes are all fitting as well if not better than they did when I was 235, so clearly the weight gain is the right type of gain. Next week I will be doing measurements to make sure everything is on the right track. This week will be another three strength-training sessions (lower body today, upper body Wednesday, and total body Friday), four days of cardio, and three days of my sorry attempt at yoga.

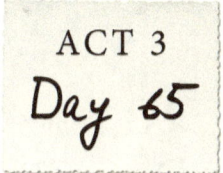

ACT 3

Day 65

Oh the joy of trying new food with a sensitive stomach: an experimental dinner I made didn't exactly agree with me. Good thing I managed to get my walk in early this morning. From what I can see I am making some good progress in changing my body even if the scale isn't moving in the right direction. Time will tell—well actually the tape will tell when I measure myself at my next weigh-in.

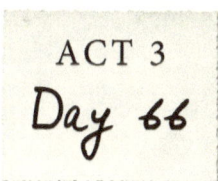

ACT 3

Day 66

Today was the second time I have done the upper body routine and I already see an increase in the amount of weight I can lift. Hopefully that keeps up. I caught a glimpse of myself in a storefront window and, dressed, I can really see the difference exercising is making; now if the scale would just cooperate. In my reading tonight I came across someone saying that it is impossible (yep, they actually said "impossible," one of my least favorite words) to gain ten pounds of muscle in a month. How can someone say that without knowing the person involved, where they started, the type of routine they were doing, their diet, or anything else? I think it is impossible to say how much muscle would be impossible to gain in any given timeframe without considering a host of variables. Not that I am saying I am going to gain ten pounds of muscle in the first month of my return to working out, but I also wouldn't declare it impossible.

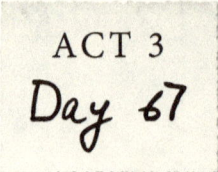

ACT 3

Day 67

Rain ruined my planned cardio day; of course I can't completely blame the weather, since I have been saying for a few weeks that I need to get indoor cardio equipment. Despite the rain we braved a dinner out to a local Italian restaurant, which I am sure will do wonders to my scale results. Italian food is one of my favorites and I know I consumed a few days worth of calories in one sitting. The next time we head out to dinner I have to pick a place with low-calorie options.

ACT 3
Day 68

A real power day today: full day of work, a good power walk, a full body strength-training routine, and an evening out all while keeping my diet in check. If only every day was as successful. I was thinking about the scale today. I am not going to worry about the number so much for the next couple weigh–ins; whatever it is, it is. After a couple weeks I will be changing my workout to a circuit-based program which essentially is moving from one exercise using light weights and doing as many repetitions as you can in one minute (each exercise is called a station) to another repeatedly doing eight to twelve exercises before taking a two minute break and then repeating the same exercises (the circuit). The benefit of a circuit routine is it can burn up seven hundred or more calories in an hour and it gives you a longer post exercise metabolism increase than traditional cardio training. Circuit workouts are the staple of many of the effective workout programs sold today and even have become a bigger part of the training routines of the military and highly conditioned professional athletes. I am designing my circuit workout myself so it might be a series of trials and errors but I am sure it will be a lot more effective than sitting on the couch. I will also lower my calorie intake for the final push that will complete this year-long journey.

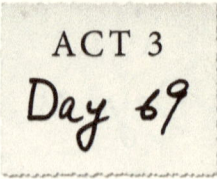

ACT 3

Day 69

Well I really countered yesterday's successes today by doing zero exercise and pigging out on a cheeseburger and onion rings. Sure I will pay for it, but every once in a while you need to let loose and enjoy life a bit; otherwise what's the point? One of those "life happens" events occurred today: as it turns out we are going to have family in town in three weeks to visit. They will only be here four days, but showing people a city like Charleston involves eating some of the finest foods, most of which do not work well with a weight loss plan. So I had to change the game plan a bit: for the next four weeks I will continue doing the same workout I have been doing: three days of strength-training, four days of cardio, and three days of yoga, and keep to a diet of around 2500 calories a day. Then for the final three weeks (once the family is out of town), I will cut the calories to 1700, add a day of cardio, and change my strength-training to a circuit-based one and hope for the best results from the final three weeks of this year-long journey.

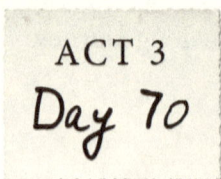

ACT 3

Day 70

I got my diet back on track and cardio done today, which is a massive improvement over yesterday. My hope is that I can have a wild day off the trail from time to time then get back on track and keep my weight under control. I decided to order two supplements: first, a good basic low-calorie protein shake and a well-respected creatine product. Obviously the protein shake serves as a meal replacement. The creatine product is supposed to aid in muscle recovery (which, trust me, I can use) and also helps promote muscle growth. We will see how these products help. Luckily we live in the modern Internet age where it is easy to research just about anything. I am not a huge fan of most supplements and I am both cautious of what I am taking and not expecting miracles. After all, they are called supplements for a reason: I expect them to supplement all the work I am doing, not do the work for me. Tomorrow is scale and measurements. I am not expecting to be too happy with either but at least I am getting on the right track; a tweak here and there and I should be ready to watch the fat fall off.

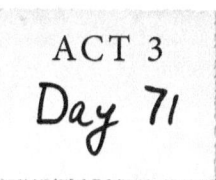

ACT 3
Day 71

MEASUREMENTS

	Start	21 Days Ago	Today	3 Week Change
Weight:	308.4	238	244.4	+6.4 pounds
Chest:	47	42	41	-1 inch
Waist:	46.5	39	38	-1 inch
Abs:	49	40	39	-1 inch
Arms:	14.5	13.5	14	+.5 inch
Thigh:	27.25	22	21	-1 inch

At first the scale number made me sick, but once I did the measurements I was a lot happier. It seems a couple weeks of working out is paying off: I am gaining weight as I lose inches, which must mean I am gaining muscle. Now I know I didn't gain six pounds of muscle in three weeks and looking at my diet over the past couple weeks I should have expected some weight gain but still the inches are moving in the right direction. The truth is the scale isn't as important as the measurements are to me at this point. I will keep trying to clean up my diet over the coming weeks but the measurements are what I am really going to focus on since, as I keep building muscles, I will hopefully be building myself a massive fat-burning machine that will allow me to eat more calories while keeping my weight in check.

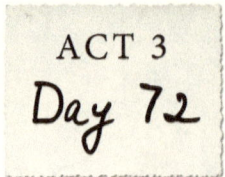

ACT 3

Day 72

Managed to get both a two-mile walk and my pathetic excuse for yoga in today despite being sore from my workout yesterday, which is enough to impress me considering how I had good excuses to do neither. I got a bit more motivation today when I put on a shirt and noticed how much better it fits now than it did a couple months ago when I went to Michigan. Even though the scale may not be lower, I am definitely smaller in the right places than I was then. Just goes to show you the scale isn't all-powerful.

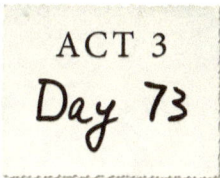

ACT 3

Day 73

Despite feeling like I got run over by a train today I managed to get my upper body workout in. Maybe the lack of sleep over the past couple days and all the working out is catching up to me because today was a tough one. It took me a while just to get myself to exercise, but once I got rolling I felt much better and was even able to increase my weights and repetitions. Hopefully tomorrow I have a bit more energy.

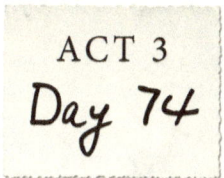

ACT 3

Day 74

I got a good yoga session in today; it is amazing how quickly you improve your flexibility. I also got my third cardio session in so only one more due this week, which means I can increase the distance and still have time to recover. My new protein powder and creatine came in today. I will have to test out the creatine to see if my stomach can handle it and to see if I get any measurable results. Based on what I read it can take seven to fourteen days to feel the effects so we will have to wait and see if it is worth the money or just another empty promise of the supplement industry. The effects I am expecting are a slight increase in muscle mass and, more importantly, a decrease in the time it takes to recover. If I get those two it's worth the money.

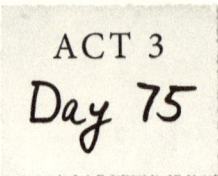

ACT 3

Day 75

Well I got a good full-body workout today. I was able to increase both the repetitions and the weight so obviously I am making progress. I also took my first two rounds of creatine today; one right after my workout and one right before bed. So far my stomach can handle it; let's hope that keeps up and the results show up sooner rather than later. Somehow I survived a trip to the grocery store, and you know they don't make it easy. I desperately needed to get more food into the house because the worst thing to do is to skip meals as that leads to weight gain and, in the long term, slows down your metabolism, which will lead to even more weight gain.

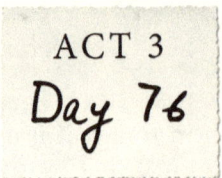

ACT 3

Day 76

I was smart enough today to take advantage of one of the most beautiful days we have had in a while and got a 2.5-mile walk in. I switched up where I walk a bit to try to keep it interesting. Also had one of the greatest rewards of weight loss today: I went clothes shopping. Today I was even able to buy a couple polo shirts in a size medium! Sure, they run a little big, but fitting into a size I haven't since my freshman year of high school got me to buy three of them. Tonight we went to a sixty-fifth birthday party and someone I haven't seen in a while actually called me skinny. Now, I am far from skinny but compared to the last time they saw me I am a lot smaller. I managed to eat right despite being at a proper southern party. I had a protein shake before we left the house, brought a protein bar with me, kept my eating at the party light (a couple rolls, some crackers and peanuts), and drank plenty of water.

ACT 3
Day 77

This is my third day on the creatine and so far I can say it makes me pee, and pee a lot. The product label says it takes seven to fourteen days to see real results; so far I've got the pee thing going on and my muscles seem to be recovering a little quicker and there's a slight increase in energy throughout the day. As the product instructs I have taken my water consumption up to 120 ounces a day, so hopefully I see more muscle size and definition and better workouts in the coming days. The taste of the product is horrible, so the results better be worth it!

ACT 3
Day 78
Weight: 242.4

Loss to date Act Three: 4 pounds

Eleven weeks in and down four pounds: isn't that just great? No wonder people jump off the weight loss wagon once dropping those pounds becomes more and more of a struggle. So what to do? Well, the first place to start is diet, so I am going to be very critical of my diet over the next week to make sure I am not only eating the right things at the right time but also not eating too many calories. Second, I am going to keep my exercise up, three days of weights, three days of flexibility, and four days of cardio a week. Third, I am going to make sure I get plenty of sleep and rest between workouts. Lastly, I am going to do my best to keep my attitude up and keep faith in this weight coming off if I continue to do the right things (I believe this will be the hardest part). Today I got the ball rolling in the right direction by walking 2.5 miles, doing my scheduled strength–training, and keeping my calories in check. Now if I can only manage to get that "faith in future results."

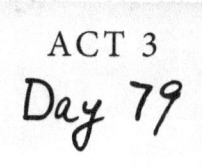

ACT 3

Day 79

I combined a good day of eating with both yoga and cardio. One "secret" to workout success I have discovered is to get two of my four weekly cardio sessions in on Monday and Tuesday; that way I can take Wednesday and Sunday off. My workweek tends to snowball, so I usually have more free time earlier in the week. In addition there is a huge sense of relief that comes from being halfway done two days into the week. I haven't been on the creatine long enough to give an honest review, but I do think my muscles are recovering a bit quicker, and of course there is still the endless amount of peeing. I have to admit I am looking forward to taking my measurements next week. I really want to see if the results I am seeing are for real or just my imagination. (Maybe creatine causes hallucinations?)

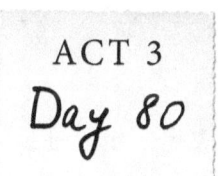

ACT 3

Day 80

Maybe I am getting results already from the creatine because I was really able to increase the weights in my upper body workout today! I really like the results I am starting to see, although there is still plenty of fat covering up my hard work. Another day of good eating combined with a good workout; the pounds ought to be flying off, right? Right? I hope to God that's right.

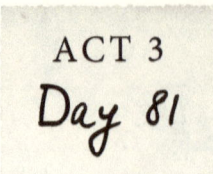

ACT 3

Day 81

A lack of sleep and a long workday makes for some serious butt dragging during workouts. Today was one of those butt-dragging days. I was able to get through both my cardio and my yoga, and I can see improvements in my flexibility. I can almost touch my toes, which is a big improvement considering a year ago I could barely see them. Once I was able to get myself out to walk I was fine; the tough part was getting going. One thing I really have to work on is getting enough sleep to make it through my now even more demanding day, so it's off to bed early and hoping tomorrow is a bit less of a struggle.

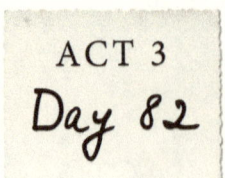

ACT 3

Day 82

Today was an adventure. We went to a town festival today, which is much like a county fair: arts, food, crafts, food, entertainment, food, you get it. I managed to avoid the food, but I went so long without eating that I was sick to my stomach from starvation by the time we got home (should have just had some funnel cake and a deep-fried candy bar if I was going to be sick anyways). We found some amazing new seasonings, which is essential when you eat chicken every day. We ended up with five new seasonings, so at least we can have a bit of variety. By the time I got to my workout I was really dragging, but I did make it through a full-body weight-training session and noticed a nice improvement despite not feeling anywhere near one hundred percent. Tomorrow I have to get my cardio and yoga in so that I can take Sunday completely off and get ready for another week.

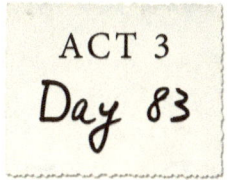

ACT 3

Day 83

Today I could really feel the effects of all the hard work I have been doing. My energy, strength, and flexibility have all improved significantly, my clothes are feeling looser, and I have some resemblance of muscle on my flabby frame. The real change is in what I call my functional fitness, which is my ability to do normal things without breaking into a massive sweat or needing a break every ten minutes. Today I managed to knock out my cardio, followed by mowing the lawn, followed by knocking out a couple items on the honey-do list, all without breaking a serious sweat. That is an awesome benefit: increased functional fitness so I can get more out of my life.

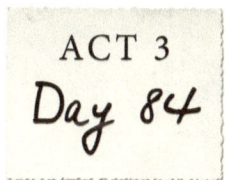

ACT 3

Day 84

Today was my rest day, so I spent a few hours working on that growing honey-do list, then spend a few hours spooning with my remote on the couch. All in all, I would call today a wash. The diet is still good and the exercise was really good this week so I am really anxious to see what the numbers look like tomorrow. I am bracing myself for a higher number than I want on the scale but improvements on the tape measure. To be frank, if I had to choose between a scale reduction and an improvement in my measurements, I would absolutely take the measurement improvement. However, let's hope I get both tomorrow morning.

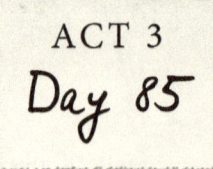

ACT 3

Day 85

MEASUREMENTS

	Start	14 Days Ago	Today	2 Week Change
Weight:	308.4	244.4	242.6	-1.8 pounds
Chest:	47	41	41	same
Waist:	46.5	38	37	-1 inch
Abs:	49	39	38	-1 inches
Arms:	14.5	14	14.5	+.5 inch
Thigh:	27.25	21	21	same

Well, the scale decided to stay the same as it was last week but at least the tape measure gave me some good results. It is tough to keep giving a hundred percent when the results don't seem to come fast enough. Sure I am looking a lot better but when you're working out to the point of nearly passing out, you expect better results. Looking back at the last couple weeks, there are only two areas I can see room for improvement (oddly enough the same two areas that always seem to need improvement for me): sleep and diet (I am eating too many carbohydrates). Over the next couple weeks I will again try to fix both of those things and hope for better results.

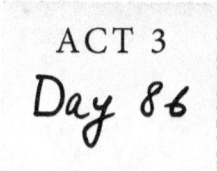

ACT 3
Day 86

Today I tried to get my unrealistic expectations to line up with the reality of my situation, realizing that I will be a work in progress for some time to come. We get such distorted body image ideas from advertisements and the media that it makes it hard to recognize the success we have had once we do lose a good amount of weight. There is no denying I look better, feel better, and am healthier than I was a year ago and that should be enough. I did manage to get a good three and a half miles in today; hopefully I can keep it up and get the scale to show me some love.

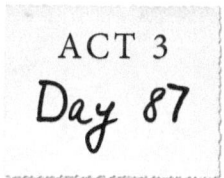

ACT 3
Day 87

Today was a challenging day: I had a full day of work and a dinner meeting but still managed to get my upper body workout in. It does get easier to fit in the workouts once you get used to the fact that you have to do them and keep the time requirement reasonable. I was able to go from start to post-workout protein shake in forty minutes. I can testify that going with basic old-fashioned weight-training gives you the greatest results in the shortest work-outs. Since you are using all free weights, you are engaging a lot more of your muscles in every exercise, which will cause the greatest muscle growth; as a bonus there is just something cool about pushing around old-fashioned weights.

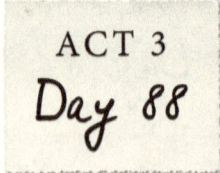

ACT 3

Day 88

I opted to skip my usual day of cardio today; the tank is beyond empty, so I need a day off to refuel. It was a day of running around like a headless chicken so I am sure I burned a few calories that way, and I did treat my dog to a walk. Fighting an eighty-five pound pit bull for a mile is a workout in itself. I remember reading a study that concluded there is no difference over time of exercising one hundred percent of the scheduled times and ninety percent of the scheduled times, so skipping a day or two shouldn't do too much damage to my progress.

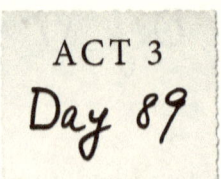

ACT 3

Day 89

I got partially back on track today. I got my full body workout in and walked the dog again but no real cardio since I am still not feeling all that great. Although I was barely able to increase the weights this workout, I was happy to get it done. I wonder if the creatine is doing more damage than good or if I just have been overworking myself. Researched some different supplements; the temptation to give in to one of the "quick fix" products out there is strongest when you are not seeing results quickly enough. Although I know at best these are empty promises and at worse they can be extremely dangerous options, the temptation is still there. Thankfully I was able to do enough research to beat into my head that I should continue to avoid them and stick with creatine and protein, but the temptation will be there until I am finally happy with my body—assuming that ever happens.

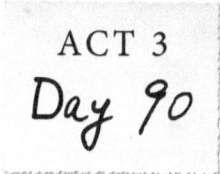

ACT 3

Day 90

I got right back on track today with cardio and yoga. The yoga was a good idea since my shoulder has been killing me; it actually kept me up last night. After I did the yoga, which I haven't done much this week, my shoulder felt amazingly better, so hopefully I remember to keep doing it since it is a lot easier than being kept awake with shoulder pain. My diet over the past two days has been outstanding: a couple real meals and protein shakes, which will hopefully make up for a couple bad meals this week come Monday's trip to the scale. Tomorrow my house gets invaded with visiting family so it will be four days of feeding them foods I shouldn't be eating and showing them a town full of food options, which again, I shouldn't be eating. I wonder how this is going to end up?

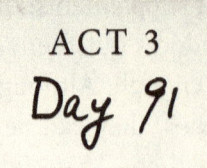

ACT 3

Day 91

The first day of the family invasion went pretty well. Luckily they came in late so it was a nice dinner at home. I had the joy of seeing some people who are still amazed by my weight loss, and one asked me a rather interesting question. When I told her I still wanted to lose more weight, she questioned if I was looking for perfection. Clearly I am far from perfection; I can't even see the outline of the perfection horizon from where I am. Though she made a good point: I do need to remember to focus on the success I have had as well as the progress I still have to make.

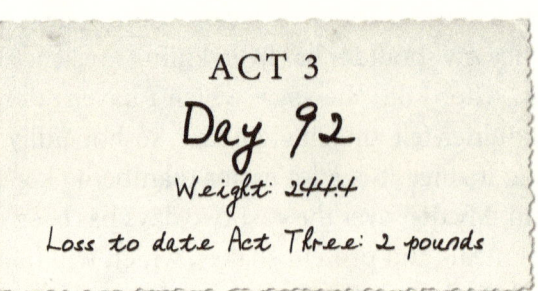

ACT 3

Day 92

Weight: 244.4

Loss to date Act Three: 2 pounds

Well I am getting bigger; hopefully it's muscle going on quicker than fat is coming off but I won't know that for another week when I do measurements again so for right now all I got is a scale moving in the wrong direction. At this point my only options are to get really strict on my diet and change my workout routines to focus more on high-calorie-burning circuit-training. I was able to squeeze out forty-five minutes between tour guide duties to get my workout in and hopefully work off some of that lunch I shouldn't have had; one can hope. The best I can really hope for out of this week is to keep my workouts up and see no upward movement on the scale, then it's three weeks to go before I have been at this for a year.

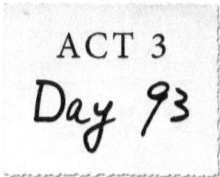

Today was far from a success. I ended up eating out poorly twice with our visiting family and didn't get any exercise in at all. Good thing our guests are only staying a couple days. I should be better at eating out by now, but I guess I still have a lot to learn.

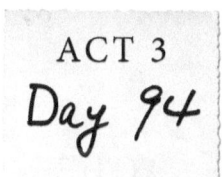

Today I took control: we did our dining at home so I could control what I was stuffing down my throat, and I got back on the exercise track, increasing the weights on every routine in my upper body workout. Interestingly I got a call from a friend who asked me if I would help him put together an exercise and nutritional program. Like me, he is a big fan of food as well as spending quality time on the couch, but he is in his mid-sixties and has had heart issues, so his program will have to be much different and he will need his doctor to approve any suggestions I give him. Although he does have some limitations, his expectations are realistic: he basically wants his pants to fit and to be able to enjoy playing with his grandkids. I could learn a thing or two from him about keeping realistic expectations considering how much I have continued to criticize myself despite others congratulating my success.

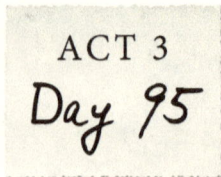

ACT 3
Day 95

Our company left today and my waistline is grateful. From their visit I learned it is very important to retain control over your diet at all times: one less meal out would have saved me enough calories to make a difference. Looking back, I also made the mistake of skipping my cardio and yoga, only managing to find time to do weight–training, so I will have to work on that as well. It is amazing how important discipline is to a healthy lifestyle.

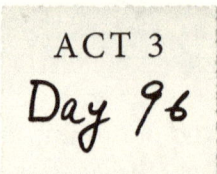

ACT 3
Day 96

I did my whole-body workout today, the absolute last of this routine since I am starting a new routine next week for my final three-week push. I wasn't feeling one hundred percent but I did get it done and sometimes that is all you can ask, especially when you are trying to catch up on a week's worth of work when you lose time playing tour guide. Tomorrow we are hitting the local farmers' market and I can't wait; this will be my first trip ever to a farmers' market, so I want to see what it's all about.

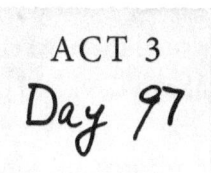

ACT 3
Day 97

Farmers' markets rock! Seriously, get yourselves to one ASAP. Today was my first but won't be my last; in fact, we will be making this a weekly event. So much fresh—and I mean right off the farm fresh—fruits and vegetables, as well as great advice on how to prepare them and, to top it all off, fantastic prices; what more can we ask for? After the farmers' market we went to the mall and I am proud to say I am now a true size-36 jean regardless of brand, as long as they aren't those skinny jeans—let's face it, skinny will never be a word to describe me or anything I might fit into. I also tried on a couple suits and I have a bit more work to do to get into a 42-long so I better make the most out of the coming twenty-one days.

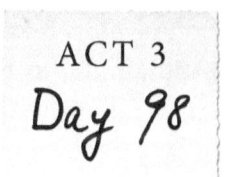

ACT 3
Day 98

Tomorrow is scale and measurement day and the start my final three-week push. I took today off both to prepare for tomorrow and to finish recovering from our house guests; I mean, they are my in-laws and after a few days of in-laws crashing at your house I think recovery is required to preserve your sanity. Let's just hope my recovery didn't do too much damage to my results.

THE FINAL THREE-WEEK PROGRAM

So what is the plan for the final three weeks?

Diet: three protein shakes a day (200 calories each), the regular meals (lean chicken or turkey, with vegetables and Greek yogurt mixed in), my nightly cup of probiotic-infused yogurt, one cup of coffee a day, at least 100 ounces of water a day, and plenty of green tea. I also am incorporating "free" foods in the form of fresh fruits and vegetables because what's healthier than fresh fruits and vegetables? My total calorie intake should be right around 2000 a day.

Exercise: I am changing my weight-training to a circuit-based training, which means doing as many repetitions as you can, with perfect form, of eight to ten exercises for a minute each, moving from one exercise to another at a quick pace. It should still take no longer than forty-five minutes but I will be moving less weight and doing more repetitions during that time. I will be working my entire body each session and doing three sessions a week. Three days a week I will be walking with some running mixed in; three times a week I will be doing yoga. This program is all about leaning out, which is the main focus for the final three weeks.

Sleep: I have to make sure I get as close to eight hours of sleep a night so my body is functioning at its best.

Desired results: I am still aiming to fit in size-34 pants and a size-42-long suit jacket, and as far as the scale, I will take any number under 235. Over the next three weeks I also want to shed two inches from my waist and abs, an inch from my chest, half an inch from my thighs, and gain half an inch on my arms. Wow, when I re-read that, I see I clearly have a lot of work to do!

ACT 3

Day 99

MEASUREMENTS

	Start	14 Days Ago	Today	2 Week Change
Weight:	308.4	242.6	242.4	-2 pounds
Chest:	47	41	41.5	+.5 inch
Waist:	46.5	37	38	+1 inch
Abs:	49	38	39	+1 inches
Arms:	14.5	14.5	14.5	same
Thigh:	27.25	21	21	same

Well somehow in the past two weeks I have managed to expand myself despite nearly exhausting myself. If I knew this was going to be the results I would have spent the past two weeks on my couch, remote in hand and pizza in mouth. Clearly I have a real challenge ahead of me over the next three weeks. Today I began my circuit-training and, let me tell you, I really need to improve my endurance. The thing with circuit-training is you don't lift real heavy weights, but you move very quickly through each exercise. The heavy weight-training I have been doing was a lot easier. My diet today was perfect: nothing to drink but water & green tea, three protein shakes, two meals of lean chicken wrapped in lettuce with Greek yogurt and a tomato on the side, and my nightly yogurt with fresh strawberries. One day down, twenty to go; the results better be a lot better than what I managed to accomplish over the past two weeks.

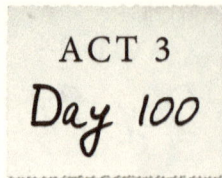

ACT 3

Day 100

As usual, day two of a new routine sucked as much as day one. Today I did a quick-paced two-mile walk and yoga, which is much easier than my circuit routine from yesterday but still sucked. It is the degree of food deprivation that likely gets to me over the first couple days; it is kind of like a lard detox that I suffer through for two to three days. My plan is to avoid the scale for another couple days, and then on day four, when I am ready to break, I will hop on and see what the results of my efforts are. Thanks to the web I found a couple much-needed replacements for my circuit routine. Hopefully I can do these without risking hospitalization; tomorrow will tell.

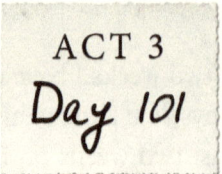

ACT 3

Day 101

Well I can report the sucking of the first two days continued through day three. For the second time the circuit-training kicked my butt. I was able to replace one of the stations and modified another to create a routine I can struggle through. Over the past three days I have noticed some subtle changes in my body and how my clothes fit but we will have to wait a few more days to see what the scale has to say (of course this could just be the result of shortage of oxygen to my brain caused by the circuit-training).

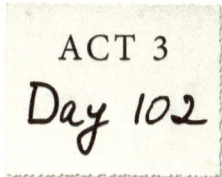

ACT 3

Day 102

Day four and the sucking continued. I took the day off from cardio today, since my circuit training is cardio as well—oh, and I can barely get up the stairs at this point. Although I took it light today, I did get my yoga in, which I hope helps with the aches and pains this week has brought. Oddly enough I was asked weight loss advice from someone my wife and I met tonight (she goes out of her way to bring up my weight loss; I think she is prouder of it than I am). It is still weird to have people ask me for my help in this arena, although I can totally understand because if someone had just dropped a bunch of weight I would have loved to get their input before I started.

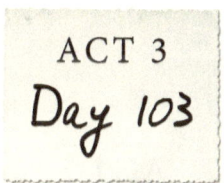

ACT 3

Day 103

Made a minor adjustment today: I did cardio instead of the circuit weight-training to give my aching shoulder a rest. Since paying my mortgage requires me to spend six to ten hours in front of a computer a day, the last thing I need is pain running from my fingers up to my shoulder blades. So I have two days to get in one weight-training session and one cardio session before the week is up; that shouldn't be a problem. Off to the farmers' market tomorrow for more fresh fruit and vegetables, which I continue to consider "free" foods—no healthy diet would deprive you of the healthiest things you can eat!

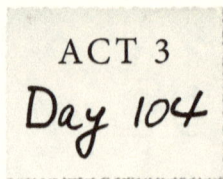

ACT 3

Day 104

Another great Saturday at the farmers' market; I can't believe I didn't start going to these things sooner! After the market, and before I rewarded myself with a healthy dose of farm-fresh strawberries, I again struggled through the circuit workout. We will have to see what the scale says Monday, but when combining the strict diet and the amount of huffing, puffing, and sweating I am doing during my workout, I expect some fantastic results. Today I also introduced another "free" food to my diet: walnuts. Walnuts are high in Omega-3 fatty acids, vitamin E, B vitamins, fiber, and protein. So my diet is lean protein and turkey, protein shakes, egg whites, all the vegetables, fruits, and walnuts I can eat, green tea, and water. If I don't see some awesome results on Monday, then I really don't know what else to do.

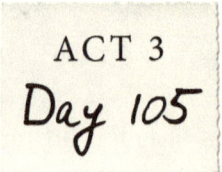

ACT 3

Day 105

Well, over the past two days I have felt a huge increase in energy. I think my body is adjusting, and starting to like my new diet and exercise routine. Today I knocked out a really well-paced three-mile walk, so hopefully that translates into an impressive result on the scale tomorrow. I have a busy week ahead of me so I am going to call it an early night and pray for the scale to move my way in the morning.

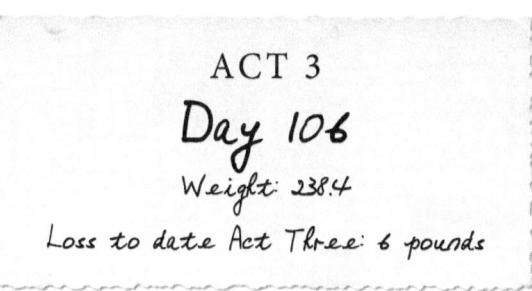

ACT 3

Day 106

Weight: 238.4

Loss to date Act Three: 6 pounds

Lost four pounds this past week, so this diet and exercise stuff actually works; who knew? Those four pounds helped motivate me through my circuit training today. Amazingly, I was able to get my workout in despite spending most of the day playing IT guy (as mentioned before one of the joys of self-employment). So even with a jammed and stressful day I still fit in a workout that kicked my butt, and I kept to the diet.

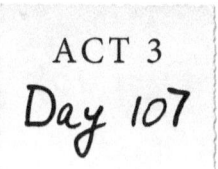

ACT 3

Day 107

Well today the diet express train ran into the brick wall that is the combination of spending too much time downtown, starving, and the comfort and ease of being able to slide into a booth at one of my favorite eateries. I figured since I was wandering off the path I might as well make it worth it: I ordered a chicken cheesesteak with sweet potato fries. Sure there were better options on the menu, but I figured if I was going to break then make it worth it. I did burn a lot of calories running around today so hopefully it won't do too much damage; hey, we all know sometimes life just happens. Besides it was just one meal; how bad can that be?

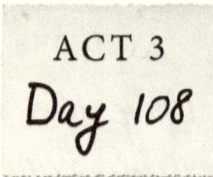

ACT 3

Day 108

I really paid for my bad eating yesterday. I must warn you that once your body gets use to a diet of lean proteins and fresh fruits and vegetables, it has a really hard time digesting less healthy options. As an added bonus I had one of those highly stressful workdays, so I really struggled through my circuit workout. So far this week I haven't done a single cardio or yoga session, and I only have four days left to get three sessions of each in; that will be a stretch since Sunday is my birthday. Happy birthday: skip the cake, go for a power walk, and hit the yoga mat!

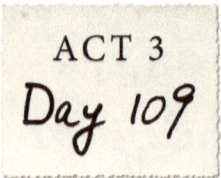

ACT 3

Day 109

Felt like a million bucks today. Even with a stressful morning of work I had endless energy. I think I worked off all the bad food from the other day, and the generous bowl of watermelon I had last night helped as well. Seriously, based on today I would say watermelon may deserve to be considered a super food because I went through the day like I had an espresso IV hooked up. Got a three-mile speed walk in, even ran a bit of it, which is always a gamble with a bad ankle and knee. But I came back in one piece, finished the night with some yoga and another heaping bowl of watermelon, and I'm ready to take on tomorrow!

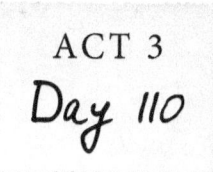

ACT 3

Day 110

Another long stressful workday, but at least today had some rewards to it. Really got a full workout in; I was drenched with sweat and gasping for air. I checked out some pictures we took the other day where I was wearing a T-shirt in public for the first time in two decades and let me tell you I am looking pretty good. I won't be flexing on the cover of a fitness magazine anytime soon, but I can pull off a T-shirt in public, which is a major accomplishment considering it has been twenty years since that was the case.

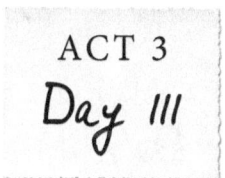

ACT 3

Day 111

So how do I unwind from a long stressful week? Well today I picked power walking through a 5K, yoga, and crashing early in the evening on my couch. Sure I was tempted to recharge by pigging out like I would a year ago, but I am sure my choice was a lot smarter. My 5K time was pretty good, and again I managed to run a small bit of it so I should have achieved a pretty good calorie burn. When combined with another good day of dieting, this should get me some good results in a couple days.

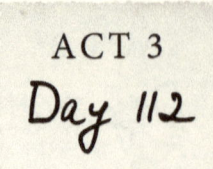

ACT 3
Day 112

Happy birthday to me, happy birthday to me—too bad you can't put a candle on a protein shake; maybe I can put one on a pear. Since today is my birthday I am splurging a bit and having homemade barbeque chicken pizza for dinner but I will wait for the cake until my year is up. It is amazing how quickly a time flies by; in eight days I will have been working for a year on my health and weight and I must say I have learned a lot—mostly through my mistakes. Let's hope I get an extra birthday present in the form of a favorable scale number tomorrow.

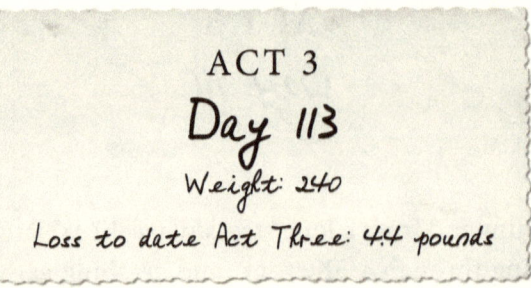

ACT 3
Day 113
Weight: 240
Loss to date Act Three: 44 pounds

Well last week surely didn't go as planned; it seems like I did a lot of work to gain 1.6 pounds in a week. Going over my weekly food log, I found a few potential reasons why the scale moved the wrong way. First, I had two bad meals and one of them was yesterday, when I had a double helping of homemade barbeque chicken pizza. Second, I started eating peanuts again around the middle of the week (hey, my wife picked them up at the grocery; all I did was fill my mouth with them—so clearly it is her fault). Third, I need to reduce the size of my midnight bowl of yogurt. I also need to start getting more than five hours of sleep a night. On the upside I know where my problems are; on the down side I only have one week left before my year-long experiment ends. For this week I am keeping my workout goals at three circuit workouts, three cardio sessions, and three sessions of yoga. My diet focus this week will be much more strict: I am going to reduce my nightly yogurt, avoid peanuts, and have fresh fruits as my between-meal snacks. I also plan on getting six to seven hours of sleep a night; mission accomplished for day one of the final week. Based on my reading and experience over the past year I firmly believe our bodies have set weights at which they naturally settle and it takes massive effort to move beyond those numbers. My body seems to love the 238- to 240- pound range. This week I plan on applying a massive effort to break through this natural plateau; let's see if my efforts work!

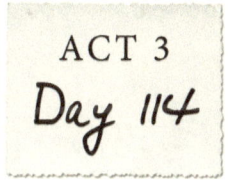

ACT 3

Day 114

Today tested my resolve about this being about health and not weight. My stomach was killing me from my workout yesterday; I really overworked my abs, so I had to give my body a rest, despite not having many days left. I know that skipping one workout won't make a dramatic difference on the scale, and more importantly it is about my health: there is nothing healthy about making a pain worse. Had it just been a bit of soreness, I would have pushed through it but this year has taught me how to recognize the difference between soreness and real pain. Hard day at work, good diet; hopefully that will be enough.

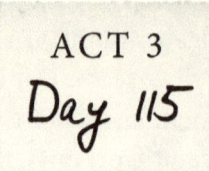

ACT 3

Day 115

I decided to take another day off from exercise to allow for a bit more healing. If you don't listen to your body, it will just talk louder and louder until you have no choice. Four days to go: I will probably get in three sessions of yoga and cardio and probably only one more session of weight-training. I also stopped taking the creatine just in case it was causing my stomach problems. Taking off and, more importantly, keeping off over seventy pounds in a year is nothing to laugh at (seriously, not a lot of laughs, some tears, a few painful groans, but really not many laughs along the way). At this point I have established exercise as a regular part of my life and have learned how to eat healthier, reversing a thirty-seven-year pattern. That's a lot to get out of one year.

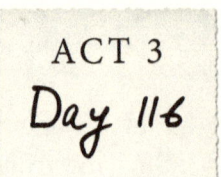

ACT 3

Day 116

My stomach felt a bit better today; hopefully the pain is just the result of me pushing too hard during my strength-training. I took it easy today: a two-mile walk and some yoga, and I feel okay. I also did a good amount of yard work today; it is still amazing how much easier those things are to do than they were a year ago. It is nice to be able to burn calories doing something other than structured exercise. Hopefully my stomach continues to improve and I can get another weight-training session in before this final week is up.

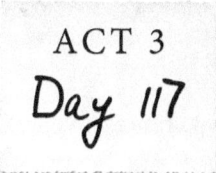

ACT 3

Day 117

Tough workday today, so I increased the cardio to 3.6 miles of fast-paced walking. I think I was trying to stomp out the day's frustration. Hey, there is a major change to note from a year ago: instead of eating to deal with frustration I power walked. I've got to say I never thought that would be the case. Another good day of dieting; positive results are in the bag.

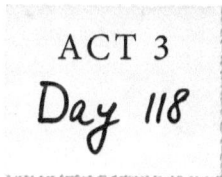

ACT 3

Day 118

With two days left, I took today off from the exercise routine to spend time around town with my wife. I figured I would burn just as many calories walking around an art festival and a farmers' market as I would around my neighborhood. I went prepared so I stuck with my diet. I keep taking my picture so I can see the success I have made, rather than focusing solely on what more I want to accomplish. I strongly suggest doing the same; if you are like me it will take a while to get used to what you look like now. The pictures help show you the success you have had so far, which should help moving you toward your long-term goals.

ACT 3

Day 119

Well the last day; tomorrow makes a year. So I did it all: walked three miles, did a new circuit workout I came up with that focused solely on the upper body, and did yoga, all in the hopes of maximizing my results tomorrow. Of course the numbers tomorrow don't matter as much as the fact that I have successfully changed my lifestyle to integrate exercise and eat a healthier diet. Early night tonight; of course I am tired considering all the exercise I did today, and the earlier I get up the earlier I get to check the numbers.

ACT 3

Day 120

MEASUREMENTS

	Start	3 Weeks Ago	Today	3 Weeks Change	Year Change
Weight:	308.4	242.4	236.8	-5.6 lbs	-71.6 lbs
Chest:	47	41.5	43	-4 in	-4 in
Waist:	46.5	38	35.5	-11 in	-11in
Abs:	49	39	38	-11 in	-11in
Arms:	14.5	14.5	15	+.5 in	+.5 in
Thigh:	27.25	21	21	-6.25 in	-6.25 in

Wow what a difference a year makes. I tried on a size-42-long suit today, and it fit, but I still need to lose a bit more to get into the size-34 pants. I am amazed at the amount of inches I have shed: eleven inches off my waist; that's insane! At the end of act one I was right about the same weight, but I was a lot bigger: my jeans were bigger and my suits were a size-46-long. Now I have to replace those suits with ones two sizes smaller. This really shows how the scale isn't the only factor to consider, since being the same weight but smaller means I put on muscle and shed body fat. As long as I keep doing that I really don't care what the scale says. Oddly enough I had a protein shake for breakfast this morning, even though my year is up and I am on a "break." From my prior breaks I have learned to control how far I let myself wander off the diet, to keep exercising, and to make sure the hiatus isn't too long.

CHAPTER SEVEN

LESSONS LEARNED

LESSONS LEARNED OVER ACT THREE AND THE LAST YEAR

What a difference a year makes. The eleven inches off my waist is more shocking that the seventy-plus pounds lost, because that is like dropping a basketball from my midsection! Some things that I learned over the past year:

- Diet is mostly responsible for simple weight loss, but transforming your body isn't just about weight loss. It takes exercise and weight-training in particular to decrease body fat and increase lean muscle mass, which both really change the way your body looks in a positive way.

- Losing weight is a lot easier than keeping weight off. You always hear people say they want to lose pounds, but what is really important is keeping those lost pounds off. Losing weight is easy, especially if you're very overweight or obese like I was when I started. A few changes in your diet and some exercise and the weight flies off. However, keeping that weight off is not only harder, since you won't see the high number of pounds falling off the scale, but also much more important to maintaining your overall health. Make sure your efforts aren't wasted and be prepared with a program to maintain your weight loss; make your goal to lose and keep off the pounds you want gone.

- At some point the scale becomes less important than the way you look, the way clothes fit, and your measurements.

- Changing your thoughts about food is difficult but very possible. In Act One, I used a preset meal plan that had me running on 700 to 900 calories a day. While this is a great way to jumpstart your weight loss and gives you time to reset your thoughts about food, it isn't sustainable (besides, who wants to live on bars and shakes the rest of their lives!). Real foods are the way to go: fruits, vegetables, lean proteins, and, yes, even some carbohydrates are all not only good for you but they taste good too. What more could we ask for!

- Do not stop exercising. Seriously, one of the big mistakes I made this year was giving myself a "break" from working out. Here is what I discovered: if you stop exercising your body begins to give back the gains you made in about a week. After a couple weeks off, you will notice really negative effects. After three weeks, your body has completely adjusted to not exercising and beginning again will be just like starting new. So even if you tone down your workouts, keep at it so you don't have to restart the wheel like I had to repeatedly.

- Allow yourself breaks in the diet routine. In reality, diets suck. Think about it: anything that restricts your ability to have something you enjoy sucks. So build breaks into your schedule. Give yourself a week or two off from time to time;

I would say no more than three weeks (as I learned the hard way), otherwise you will have too much ground to make up. However, a couple weeks off can be just enough to recharge your batteries and get you ready to go at it again.

- Supplement with care. Remember, supplements can *at best* offer a slight assist to the hard work you do. If your diet is bad, no supplement will take weight off; if you don't exercise, no supplement can put muscle on. From my readings, it seems a lot of supplements can be downright dangerous so take caution and review your supplement choices with your doctor and not just the guy working behind the supplement store counter.

- Focus on the progress you have made, not just how far you are from your goal. After a year of hard work I still have about twenty-five pounds of fat I want to lose and another ten pounds of muscle I want to add, but that goal is nowhere near as important to my general health as the seventy pounds and eleven inches off my waist I already dropped. Keep yourself positive and on the right path by focusing on the success you have along the way and not just the work you still have in front of you.

- Sleep is essential. This is a hard one for me; I tend to sleep four to five hours a night, but typically you need seven hours for your body to have proper time to repair itself.

- Learn to listen to your body. Know the difference between sore (expected from strenuous exercise), hurt (noticeable pain when using, needs to be rested), and injured (continual noticeable or limiting pain, needs medical attention). You also need to develop a good working relationship with your doctor so you can ensure everything you do along your journey is in the best interest of your overall health.

- Circuit-training is great for those of us battling extra weight. It can burn a lot more calories than almost any other exercise in thirty to forty-five minutes. It is also great for those of us with existing joint issues because you are using much lighter weights. The basics of circuit-training are simple: group eight to twelve exercises (stations), do each for one minute (typically around thirty reps) with lighter weights; move from one station to the next until all stations have been done once (that is a circuit), take a two-minute break, and repeat one or two more times.

- Vary your workout routines. Your body adjusts quickly, typically in about three weeks, to whatever you throw at it, so have a couple different types of cardio and a couple different workout routines in your back pocket to throw your body a curveball and keep the losses coming.

- Don't get caught up beating yourself up when you slip up. Everyone has bad days, lazy days and downright wasted days so you're not alone. You don't need to beat yourself up about it, accept it, realize why you did it, and make sure you put an end to it. Whether it's a bad day, a rough week or a lost month move on. The past is what got you to where you are but what you do in the present is what get's you the future results you want so focus on the present and get back to it!

- Realize that fitness is a lifelong process. This journey isn't over for me, nor will it ever be. I will constantly be working to be a better version of me. If you are just starting out and can only walk a mile every other day don't get discouraged because this isn't a sprint, it's a lifelong marathon! Just increase your distance a little each week, increase the repetitions or weight you use when strength training a little each session and work each week to eat a little better than you did the last week and you will get there. Remember there is no way to get there quickly but if you dedicate yourself to making improvements over time you will exceed your goals.

SO WHERE TO GO FROM HERE?

Well, I am taking it easy for two weeks then I will have about a month before my twentieth high school reunion (again using a personally meaningful event as my target). I plan on spending that month making as much of an impact as I can. Now when I say taking it easy, I have learned that doesn't mean stop exercising and eat with reckless abandon. Taking it easy now means keep the exercise up and watch most of what I eat, but allow myself a less restrictive diet and more calories per day. These two weeks are my reward for a year of hard work, but I don't want to give back all my gains. I want to be able to get right back at it and make significant improvements in the final month before my reunion. After I return from the reunion I plan on keeping at it and eventually reaching my own goal of getting my weight under two hundred pounds, in my own time. For the first year, I think I made some real significant changes in both my body and my lifestyle. It is truly amazing what is possible when you spend a year combining hard work, sweat, and faith.

www.ingramcontent.com/pod-product-compliance
Lightning Source LLC
Chambersburg PA
CBHW022249290526
45785CB00015B/434